THE
HEALING
WISDOM
OF
AFRICA

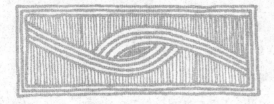

MALIDOMA
PATRICE SOMÉ

TARCHERPERIGEE
AN IMPRINT OF PENGUIN RANDOM HOUSE

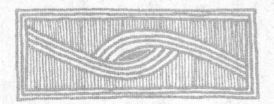

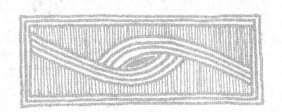

THE
HEALING
WISDOM
OF
AFRICA

Finding Life Purpose
Through Nature,
Ritual, and Community

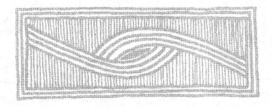

tarcherperigee

an imprint of Penguin Random House LLC
1745 Broadway, New York, NY 10019
penguinrandomhouse.com

Library of Congress Cataloging-in-Publication Data

Somé, Malidoma Patrice, date.
The healing wisdom of Africa : finding life purpose through nature,
ritual, and community / Malidoma Patrice Somé.—1st trade pbk. ed.
p. cm.
ISBN 0-87477-991-X
1. Dagari (African people)—Rites and ceremonies.   2. Spiritual healing.
I. Title.
[BL2480.D3S65   1999]   99-24829   CIP
299'.64—dc21

Printed in the United States of America

The authorized representative in the EU for product safety and
compliance is Penguin Random House Ireland, Morrison Chambers,
32 Nassau Street, Dublin D02 YH68, Ireland. https://eu-contact.penguin.ie.

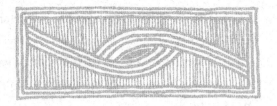

ACKNOWLEDGMENTS

This book would have never come to life without the contribution and efficacious labor of a number of people. First in the list are the ancestors and spirits whose inspiration and blessings took the form of ideas translatable into the English language. As an old wisdom would say, "The light that shows the way is a gift from loving beings in the Other World." They wrote the book.

I would like to extend my deep gratitude to Damon P. Miller II, M.D., a physician and healer who understood the idea and the importance of the material presented in this book. Without him, the torture of writing on a subject of this magnitude would have been insufferable. Dr. Miller burned considerable time and effort with the rewriting and editing of the book, even as I was feeling that the scope and the ambition of this undertaking were too great.

My sincere thanks to my wife, Sobonfu Somé, for her support and patience during the stormy days of materializing the thoughts and ideas that form this book.

I also extend my gratitude to John Strohmeier, who took time off from his busy schedule to help me straighten my often failing English.

Many thanks to my development editor, Priscilla Stuckey, who brought a much needed organization to the book, presenting the ideas in a context that makes them shine with special brilliance. Her perceptiveness and sensitivity in rewriting added the fire of vision to the manuscript, and she vigorously towed the book onto the firm land of clarity and fluidity. What I gained from the experience were the trust and friendship that allowed me to stay confident that this book would come into existence.

Finally I would like to acknowledge those publishers who permitted the use of materials.

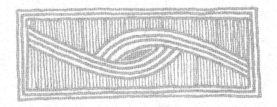

CONTENTS

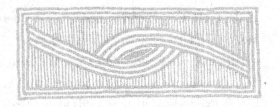

Living in Two Worlds

If you don't know the kind of person I am
and I don't know the kind of person you are
a pattern that others made may prevail in
the world and following the wrong god
home we may miss our star.

—WILLIAM STAFFORD,
"A Ritual to Read to Each Other"

My name is Malidoma. It means "he who makes friends with the stranger/enemy." I come from a little village in West Africa named Dano, located in the landlocked country of Burkina Faso. I belong to a group of people called the Dagara, who trace their origins to the region once known as the Gold Coast, now called Ghana. There are three different settlements of the Dagara people that I know of. The first, which is said to be the original, is located on the coast of Ghana. I've never been there, but I hear that anyone who wants to discover the source of Dagara magical knowledge and spirituality needs to go there.

The second settlement is in northern Ghana. Its only distinction from my own is that colonial forces artificially divided the group into two separate nationalities. A large number of tribal communities throughout the world suffered the same fate of being divided by the casual decree of colonizers. In Ghana it happened in the 1880s, in a government office somewhere in Belgium. Those who drew the boundaries did not know of, or care about, the Dagara people.

The Dagara people are well known throughout West Africa for beliefs and practices that outsiders find both fascinating and frightening. The Dagara connection with beings from the Spirit World has resulted in the accumulation of firsthand knowledge of subjects regarded in the West as paranormal, magical, or spiritual. Dagara "science," in this sense, is the investigation of the Spirit World more than the world of matter. What in the West might be regarded as fiction, among the Dagara is believed as fact, for we have seen it with our eyes, heard it with our ears, or felt it with our own hands. The stories I tell often sound, to Western ears, fantastic, for hearers lack the advantage of the comprehensive investigations into the interplay of spirit and matter that characterize the Dagara and many other African peoples.

The story of my youth and education is described in my previous book, *Of Water and the Spirit*. In it I walk the reader through a life at the edge, between two cultures, one indigenous and the other modern. The story is a tempestuous one.

I am one of a few thousand native Africans who, at an early age (four years old, in my case), were stolen from one world and taken to another as part of the European colonial project, through the efforts of the French and the Roman Catholic Church. The fascination of Dagara people with matters pertaining to Spirit particularly predisposed them to the acceptance of French Catholicism. In retrospect, I think many Dagara saw assimilation into French Catholicism much as they saw our tribal rites of initiation: the replacement of an old self with a new, in the interest of a better life. Many approached colonial religious practices with the intention of exploring them only briefly, but they soon lost their bearing, becoming acculturated and easily manipulated. My father was part of this group, bitten by the bee of curiosity only to find himself trapped. My Western education and habituation to the ways of the West at the hands of Catholic missionaries was a result of his entrapment. He had made a deal with the colonizers, a deal in which I had no say, a deal that he did not fully understand. Through this deal, I was removed from my family and village and taken to the priests' missionary school to become acculturated. Once I was gone, the pleas of my father to return me fell on deaf ears. I remained in the missionary school system until the age of twenty.

In retrospect I cannot believe how much I wanted to kill my father for delivering me into the hands of Western teachers. But that was before my acceptance of the prophecies surrounding my life. My people hold dear a view of personhood that contrasts with modern empirical thinking. The Dagara believe that everyone is born with a purpose, and that this purpose must be known in order to ensure an integrated way of living. People ignorant of their purpose are like ships adrift in a hostile sea. They are circling around. As a result, tribal practices emphasize the discovery, before birth, of the business of the soul that has come into the world. A person's purpose is then embodied in their name, thus constituting an inseparable reminder of why the person walks with us here in this world. In my case, I was meant to get involved with other cultures in the interest of redefining relationships in a spirit of harmony. Hence the name Malidoma, which means "he who makes friends with the stranger." For this reason, it feels as if I went to school not only to learn the ways of the stranger, but also to learn ways of making friends.

I have to make clear that in the years immediately following the colonial period of the 1950s and 1960s, missionary schools continued to flourish in Africa. While the Europeans who had carried bombs and guns into

West Africa were interested in material resources, those who wielded the cross were interested in souls. Thus, the purpose of these schools was clear: to continue the work of European colonization on the African continent by converting natives to Christianity and the ways of the West while they were still young, susceptible, and easy to persuade. This was not a localized program in West Africa but a widespread practice spanning the entire African continent.

School, to us, was a place where we learned to reject whatever native culture we had acquired as children and to fill its place with Western ideas and practices. This foreign culture was presented as high culture par excellence, the acquisition of which constituted a blessing. Going to school was thus a radical act involving the sacrifice of one's indigenous self. For the white Catholic missionaries who were building a Christian empire, such a project was necessary for survival, a consequence of the decline of Christian faith in Europe.

French colonial encroachment into Africa started in the latter part of the eighteenth century and increased dramatically with new conquests and settlements throughout the nineteenth century. During that time, colonial governments were manned exclusively by officials and support personnel imported from France. But by the early twentieth century, native Africans who had been educated to act on behalf of the colonizer, using the colonizers' own methods, were enlisted to maintain the prosperity of the colonial dispensation.

The two great wars of the twentieth century brought tremendous changes to the colonial empires. Among them was the opening of the eyes of the colonized regarding the fact of their colonization, resulting in the worldwide political movement known as nationalism. This real identity could be described as deceptive, exploitative, and disruptive. In Africa, young educated blacks began using the pen and podium to express their discontent. Trapped in a cultural paradox that defined them as both white and black, they could not contain their anger. On the one hand, it was impossible for them to return to their native land and ways, because a cultural barrier stood before them. This barrier was the native language that they could no longer speak and the living conditions in the village, devoid of Western amenities. On the other hand, they could not stay among Westerners and enjoy their newly acquired cultural identity, mainly because of white social and economic rejection. Consequently, they created a diaspora of struggling people adrift in the vast sea of cultural anonymity. This gave rise to what has now entered the canon of nationalistic literature known as négritude, spearheaded by figures such as Léopold Sédar Senghor, former president of Sénégal, and now a member of the French Academy. Négritude is the owning of being black in the face of white rejection of blacks.

Toward the middle of the twentieth century, under the increasing pressure of nationalist activists and the United States government, imperial European nations decided to grant independence and self-rule to their colonies. The late fifties and early sixties saw a massive birth of new nations from the bellies of European mother countries. Suddenly geographic areas that were once administered by French colonials, for example, were to be administered by black Africans trained by the French.

The first decade of leadership by these blacks was disastrous to postcolonial Africa. Many indigenous people, out of concern for themselves, began to wonder when independence was going to end. Leaders emulating the totalitarian rule of colonial administrators terrorized their own people, only to find themselves driven from power by others more zealous in the business of torturing their people and kin. Meanwhile, European countries continued to maintain strong involvements with their former colonies, exerting considerable control over the leadership that had assumed their role. In short, colonial tyranny did not leave Africa, it simply changed its face. The maintenance of colonial languages as the new countries' official ones, the literal copying of colonial political administration, and above all the strict observance of Western manners, are all elements that have combined to give birth to the Third World.

Postcolonial Africa inherited three basic languages from the West: French, English, and Spanish. These languages are its official languages, and people go to school to learn how to speak, read, write, and think in them. The governments of these countries copy the style of the country in Europe that colonized them, and the people in the official government positions act, dress, eat, sleep, and live like Europeans.

To learn new ways, to acquire a new vision to replace the old one learned in native villages, as was the mode of education in the Christian schools, meant to experience pain at the hands of angry and overzealous teachers. These teachers acted as if theirs was the most miserable job in the world, and they directed their anger and frustration at the very people they were teaching. Why were they so emotionally strained? Because these teachers were also shaped and changed by the violent methods of colonial training, and ultimately found themselves, like their students, trapped between two worlds, unable to fully participate in either.

I suspect that every literate African who went to a colonial school such as mine carries, as I do, the marks of his literacy on his body. These marks are not small scars. Literacy was literally beaten into us, and to avoid pain we had to quickly master European languages. Western knowledge finds a cozy place in the African consciousness when carefully packaged inside a whip and regularly delivered. No wonder former French president Charles de Gaulle complained that the French language was better spoken by colonial Africans than by French citizens themselves.

The grave problem related to this manner of education is that its fanaticism breeds fanaticism in the student. You can't beat someone into enlightenment without fearing that this violence will be returned to you someday. There comes a time when the young pupil begins to see cracks in the curriculum of ideology. And with the energy of adolescence comes a high level of aggressiveness which, in our case, was turned against postcolonial authority. I regret to confess that it led me at the age of twenty to hit a priest and then escape from the mission school, driven away by fear of the consequences of such an act. That fear became fuel enough to carry me all the way back to my village on foot. For other young students, responses ranged from teacher assassination to suicide. In every case it was a response to the unbearableness of cultural repression.

Because education was a departure from home and all its values, because it meant forgetting the ancestral ways in order to survive, education fostered in me and my colleagues a serious crisis of identity. When I returned to my village, the home I found was not in any way like home to me. Initially I could not accept that this was the place of my birth. Faced with blatant uncleanliness, nakedness displayed without shame, and painfully unsophisticated dwellings, I began to pity my own people. Even worse, their lack of awareness of how backward, stagnant, and uncouth they were drove me to anger at the unfairness of God for associating me with them. For the first time since being taken from home, the language I had been forced to acquire became useless, and at the same time, my native language abandoned me. People in the West may have a hard time imagining what it is like to be unable to speak one's native language, unable to communicate properly to one's own parents and family. One can only know this through experience. I learned that a homecoming can never be complete until feelings are properly communicated and shared.

My return to the village after some sixteen years of schooling at the mission school meant the beginning of my education in another culture— my own. I was not whipped by teachers this time, though this did not make the education any easier. What I noticed immediately was that native learning clashed with my previous education, creating a strange kind of commotion within me. The sensation was most interesting because my newly acquired indigenous values gradually overshadowed the concepts learned in the course of my Western education, scaring away the notion that my own culture was primitive and doomed.

At the colonial school I had been told that the rituals my people performed to heal were devilish and inspired by Satan. But I discovered that there were countless illnesses that could not be healed at the local infirmary which were perfectly curable at the hands of Dagara healers. I wondered whether saving lives was indeed devilish or satanic. At school, we had also been told that tribal people have no knowledge of magic, but instead are very superstitious. When I witnessed Dagara people make things appear and disappear into thin air, when I witnessed beings from the Other World show up in flesh and bones allowing me to touch them, I

wondered how superstitious all this was. And then there was my introduction to the *kontombli*, the spirits in the wild who worked as the com-
forter of every person in need. All of these experiences contradicted the
theories disseminated in the schools.

At the same time, it was interesting to see the reaction of villagers who
observed what literacy had done to me. I discovered that, from their perspective, what I learned from my white teachers was considered poison-
ous, and even dangerous, to me and others. It was as if literacy destroyed
the ability to learn the indigenous knowledge that I was trying to reclaim.
With literacy had come a logic that was incompatible with the logic innate
to the Dagara and other native peoples. It made me prone to doubt, incapable of trust, and subject to dangerous emotions such as anger and impa-
tience. Worst of all, my Western perceptions of time were continually
disturbing me in a culture in which timelessness prevailed.

In retrospect I now realize that I was my own worst enemy in the quest
for the magical and the supernatural. Because of the Western consciousness I had absorbed and its grandiose notions of superiority, I was slow to
accept any interference or intrusion from an indigenous worldview. It was
as if one type of knowledge had colonized my thoughts, with a territorial
instinct of the most vicious type. For example, my literacy came with a
mind that loved to affirm itself by wielding the sword of analysis. When
my mind failed to fit events into its various rational slots, it was prompt to
dismiss them as primitive trickery unworthy of civilized thinking. As long
as new knowledge did not fit the desired specifications for proper control,
my Western-trained mind regarded it as an alien with hostile intention
and therefore would fight against it with patriotic pride. I realize now that
what I thought was my civilized mind was in fact a rather narrow mind.
The knowledge I had been exposed to in Western schools left a wide
range of experience unexplored, and it was up to wise people in my village to help me learn to open up to all the realms of knowledge of which
I at that time was ignorant.

After I returned to my village, I was gently approached and carefully
nursed by my *madaba*, my "male mother," Uncle Guisso. He alone had

the dexterity to dress the wound of my psyche without provoking further hemorrhaging. In Guisso's emergency room, the vital signs of my psyche were stabilized, allowing me gradually to awaken to the realities that would help me reconcile my educated self with the culture of my ancestors. My initiation, in particular, enabled me to understand this. Initiation was a serious undertaking for both Guisso and me, an undertaking beyond the scope of this writing or any writing. At its core was the objective of restoring the damaged regions of my psyche which, as though infected by a virus, were responsible for my crisis of identity. Such a restoration required that I confront a body of realities that widened my spiritual horizons immensely, but at the same time put my life at risk. Exposure to the magical can be as dangerous to a person as exposure to high levels of radiation. Without proper protection one runs the risk of losing one's self to the very world that radiates these energies. Consequently a romantic attraction to magic is often a naive impulse toward the sacred that unveils a dangerous ignorance of what one is attracted to. I think I made it through these trials not because I was intelligent, but because my *madaba* is a gifted indigenous scientist, the kind that Westerners might call a shaman. I was fortunate. And my good fortune became even more evident when I realized the good that came with exposure to the magical world.

I call my initiation a radical healing. My angry, vicious self was quieted, intimidated by the sweeping powers of the Other World. Something like a new person was born in me. The region of my psyche that had been put to sleep at the schools of Western thought was suddenly restored. I was reconnected to the deep regions of my psyche and to all living things. I rediscovered my home in the natural world, which is the true home of all beings on earth. And I was reconciled to my family and to the village community into which I had been born. I was alive and in awe of what I felt. My indigenous life was allowed to resume.

My initiation was followed by a quiet, seemingly uneventful year in the village. I began to grow accustomed to the slow and quiet magic of the village. With the entrance of the spiritual into my psyche, I began to see why the life I was embracing—so marvelously eventful on the inside—

could be seen by a Western-trained eye as unattractive. How does one judge what cannot be seen?

But too soon, unfortunately, there came a day when my destiny overtook me. That day the village leader, the *tensob*, spoke to me about my life's purpose, intimating what I had not thought about since my return to the community. I had long suspected that "making friends with the stranger/enemy" would someday mean separation from my village and family. The village leader addressed me in the most diplomatic terms, but his words were painful, for I understood at once that I was to leave. I was being politely exiled—now, after finally finding the home that had been lost to me. The grief that ensued was a reaction to his announcement that I must return to school to master the ways of the West.

As I quieted down I was able to understand more clearly the philosophy of the Dagara elders toward the West, a philosophy of inclusiveness and flexibility shaped by an awareness that the West was here to stay. Coping with the West was better than pretending it did not exist. Wasn't the spread of literacy among the indigenous people of West Africa an irreversible manifestation of its presence? I recalled my own father innocently asking me if I could forget how to read and write in order to diminish the pain of initiation. It sounded silly at the time, but later on I discovered the depth of this simple remark. Indeed literacy is a Western condition that, once acquired, cannot be denied. Yet I remained puzzled at the idea that I could learn anywhere things that would rival the wisdom that I had learned in my own village in so short a time.

In the end, I accepted my return to school as a not entirely bad or undesirable fate. For someone whose name means "make friends with the stranger/enemy" it made sense to pursue a higher level of Western education after learning what I had learned among my people. But the thought of returning to school resurrected deeply buried fears. For me, in many ways, it was the same as going to hell. I needed major adjustments to align my thoughts with the decision of the elders. As my fears emerged, they summoned forth my power to argue. But unlike in the West where linear, rational logic enables people to argue their way in and out of situations, my best arguments were not enough to exempt me from my destiny.

Entering the University of Ouagadougou, one day's journey from my home, I felt as if I were confronting, not once again but in an entirely new way, the business of living in two worlds. The proximity to home made it possible to continue to work with my *madaba*, thereby allowing the two sources of my education to parallel each other. It felt good. The contrasts were huge and the ironies obvious. Unlike my earlier Western education, when it was impossible even to imagine that there could be two types of knowledge, now indigenous and modern were able to coexist in me without the modern surreptitiously coercing and dwarfing the other. There seemed to be a great freedom in recognizing the separate place from which my Western teachers presented their world to me. Just as knowledge from one world can help the knower live in another, I found myself constantly invoking the powers of the ancestors to navigate through school and in the Western world.

I must admit that my apprenticeship with my *madaba* was more exciting than my university studies. In the village, as in a laboratory, I could see, experience, and participate in a series of exciting secret ventures that stretched my conception of truth so widely that in the end I could not help but contrast them with the almost deliberate narrowing of reality in modern thought. Healers in the village taught that Westerners tried to control magic by insisting on knowing a visible cause for anything that might happen. This expectation had the sad and inevitable effect of mystifying rather than clarifying reality, since as village people know, different laws operate in the different dimensions of reality. A Westerner will say, for example, that water always makes you wet, yet a native healer who gets into a river and stays for hours doing what healers do might get out just as dry as if he had been working in the Sahara Desert.

Education in the West meant graduating, first from the university in Ouagadougou, then from the Sorbonne in Paris, then from Brandeis University in the United States. Each degree reflected a conception of learning that was far different from the educational experience in my village. In the schools of the West, when I graduated I received a formal document certifying that I had completed a program of difficulty and importance and was now granted the right to enjoy the privileges of my accomplishment. In the village, on the other hand, every discovery, every learning mastered, led to a far different response. The elders instead said something like, "Having been exposed to this and that and successfully endured its pain, we now grant you the right to more trouble and tribulation for your own growth and for the fulfillment of the destiny associated with you. May the ancestors continue to stay by your side."

For an African to come to the West while maintaining a devotion to ancestral wisdom is to invoke a program of challenges and adversity. Here in the West, Africa has been much written about, but in areas such as religion and spirituality, where Africa has quite a profound wisdom to contribute, it has been for the most part written off. Many Westerners have written about African spirituality, but they pay scant attention to the practices that might benefit Westerners. Most references instead discuss rather disturbing magical practices such as blood sacrifices, voodoo, and witch doctors involved with evil rituals. And in fact scores of educated Africans in positions of influence have publicly rejected the spiritual practices of their kinsfolk as primitive and barbaric.

I still remember hearing judgments ranging from "superstitious" to "savage" uttered by African leaders and intellectuals to their own people. As a consequence, I learned that showing to the world what I was learning of the vast body of native wisdom could result in a great deal of confusion and suffering. I recognized that discretion—and sometimes even deliberate deception—was necessary in order to protect myself from naive and negative criticism which can be profoundly disempowering. I used to pretend to curious outsiders that I did not know anything, to the great delight of my indigenous teachers. I would consciously make mistakes in order to protect myself and my knowledge, suggesting to outsiders that I knew very little of value.

In the West, one can find indigenous cultural elements embedded in American culture if one knows where to look for them. The widespread fascination with antiquities, adventure travel, and tribal artifacts reveals a culture hungry to connect with indigenous roots. It is only through a massive investment in denial of indigenous spirituality that many Westerners have arrived at the relatively comfortable thinking that "modern" means that which has overcome primitivism, that which is superior to the indigenous.

But just as indigenous peoples have accepted that the modern world won't go away, Westerners need to recognize that indigenous thought is here to stay as well. The indigenous world may have to be redefined by Westerners in new forms. Just as traces of the philosophy, architecture, and politics of the classical Greeks are still apparent all over the Western world in modernized forms, the ancient indigenous ways will silently continue to pervade the fabric of modernity. Indigenous wisdom is destined to continue undisturbed beneath these transformations.

When I arrived at Brandeis University I was stunned to discover how little Americans, even in academia, knew about Africa. To many, Africa consisted of three or four countries, namely South Africa, Nigeria, Kenya, and sometimes Ghana, even though to some the name Ghana sounded more like a town in South Africa than a nation in West Africa. Most Americans knew the entire continent as one large, rather insignificant, more or less unified country. They seemed to prefer it that way. They also liked to assume that many Africans slept in trees, or in more advanced rural areas, lived in thatched huts. Needless to say, few people had heard of the country of Burkina Faso, let alone knew that French is spoken there. A great many who only spoke English were amazed to discover that English is my third language. They had little or no understanding of the importance of foreign languages.

I remember a conversation in which a student, bemused by the fact that I came all the way from Africa to study at a prestigious school in America, asked if Africans preferred to sleep in trees. When I told him that, in fact, the American ambassador slept in the biggest tree in the capital, he became visibly upset with me and walked away. I also discovered that things which international students were required to know about the

West were unknown to many of my American colleagues. I felt deceived, for example, when I discovered that college students here did not know where the Four Corners region was, and that some thought that New Mexico was located somewhere in Mexico.

American students also expected me to know very little about modern culture. Because most of my fellow students had made up their minds about who, as an African, I was, they assumed I did not know such things as how to use a microwave, drive a car, or operate a washing machine. They delighted in showing me these things without first verifying that I did not know them already. I learned that in order to make people like these comprehend, let alone appreciate, ancestral culture, I would need the help of miracles.

I found here in the West people who were so submerged in the massive trance of modern culture that they appeared virtually unreachable. It became clear that certain topics of discussion, such as spirituality and rituals, were not permitted in intellectual and professional circles. I noticed some people, particularly those who were most enthralled by the game of consumerism, found mention of indigenous wisdom especially irritating and sometimes would lash out at me, just as a child entranced by a Nintendo game reacts with a tantrum to any disturbance. I am still recovering from the inflamed words of people who retaliated at me for referring to indigenous people as having power. Time and again, I have been faced with angry questions like, "If Africans are so full of wisdom, why are they shooting each other? Why can't they stop famine?"

I ask in response, "Where do these weapons come from?" Colonialism weakens a native people by, among other things, sapping its economy and creating scarcity. Everyone knows that scarcity results in the loss of human dignity. A person whose identity has been violated becomes subject to control. If a gun is then given to such a person to use as a way of restoring his sense of dignity, chances are he will use it. My people are frustrated by the lack of credibility they experience from the modern world, and many have lost hope that anything but the gun will be heard. This book is a response to and a reaction against such thinking.

Today, while most people in the West enjoy material affluence, villagers in Africa suffer hunger and poverty. But here, perhaps, is a case where the material and the spiritual are working independently toward the same end. Africa's material scarcity may be symptomatic of a deeper global problem pertaining to soul and Spirit. While the Third World is experiencing the immediacy of the people's need for healing in the area of physical hunger, the West is awakening to a spiritual hunger so dramatic as to be almost frightening. Like the famished cows in the Pharaoh's dream, the modern psyche dangles and zigzags this way and that way with a mighty intent to devour anything that smells ancient and spiritual. The converging paths of these two worlds may ultimately enable material abundance to silence the Third World body's cries for nourishment and the cries of the Westerner's hungering soul.

It became clear to me that if I was to become the friend of the stranger/enemy, it was necessary to become skilled in articulating indigenous meaning so that it might resist dismissal at the hands of modern discursive logic. I do not know if I can ever be successful at this, but I know it is a challenge that is always fresh and ready to be tackled once again.

I have gradually come to understand that one thing Western and indigenous peoples share is the fact that both have elected to live here on Earth, and are thus subject to the spirit of Earth. By this I simply mean that indigenous and Western peoples are actually children of the same Spirit, living in the same house they call Earth. No matter what they do to torture each other, the dysfunctional relationship of modern and indigenous peoples is symptomatic of a craving to share love for each other that is deeply buried in our psyches, a craving so alive that it is compelled to struggle through the rubble of division, power conflicts, and fear to express itself.

The purpose of this book is not only to promote understanding between Western and indigenous cultures but also to show how the indigenous world and its wisdom might heal many of the spiritual and emotional problems from which Western civilization suffers. Among these ills are the pervasive sense of loneliness and isolation from which many modern people suffer; the absence of a supportive community to help individuals weather the storms of life; the feeling of anonymity that results when a culture prohibits the expressing of true emotion; and the distractions of consumerism, which lead people away from focusing on the things that matter most deeply to them.

To many readers, my outline of African wisdom may appear a blatant idealization of the indigenous. The reason is simple: I am not interested in recounting all the bad things that indigenous Africans are known to do; these are abundantly available in the Western media. If this book leads you to feel that I have been unfair to the West, that the picture is not balanced, that Western culture is not given its fullest due, then perhaps you will identify with the feelings that I as an African experience when I read books written by non-Africans about Africa. This book will probably challenge your beliefs. I do not expect that you will come to agree with me on every point. But perhaps you can understand how the beliefs in this book form a coherent system for understanding the world. At the very least, the beliefs deserve a respect and reverence they seldom receive.

In this book you will not find complete recipes, prescriptions, and easily applied tools for solving modern ills. You will find instead some ways of looking at the human being and at society that you may not have considered before. My goal is not to convert you to an indigenous point of view, but to offer and recommend that view as a potential enrichment to your present life.

I remember well a conversation between a shaman and a simple villager about the relationship between the West and the indigenous world. The villager was convinced that Westerners were witches because they had mastered the power of enticing his children away. He said this because his children had abandoned the village for the city, leaving him alone.

It was not this man's observation that caught my attention, but the response of the shaman, a young man in his early thirties fully grounded in the art of healing. He said that his training had taught him that the white man came to Africa primarily to heal himself, not to steal people from the villages. He went on to say, "We Africans also believe that we need healing at the hand of the white man. This is why our children leave us. You see, it's the same world, the same house. When someone is sick, everyone is. Why should we remain passive while the white man searches the world for the means to save himself? We are together in this struggle. All our souls need rest in a safe home. All people must heal, because we are all sick."

It is possible that we have been brought together at this time because we have profound truths to teach each other. Toward that end, I offer the wisdom of the African ancestors, so that Westerners might find the deep healing they seek. From an indigenous perspective, the individual psyche can be healed only by addressing one's relationships with the visible worlds of nature and community and one's relationships with the invisible forces of the ancestors and Spirit allies. For this reason, much of the book concerns the practice of ritual, for it is in ritual that nature, community, and the Spirit World come together to support the inner building of identity.

In Part One we will look at the indigenous world and its views of healing. Part Two concerns the relationships of healing, namely those found in community. In Part Three I provide some background for understanding and engaging in the rituals, which I then outline in Part Four. I offer suggestions for developing rituals to heal the deep wounds of disconnection from Spirit and ancestors, the wounds of isolation and invisibility, the wound of stuckness in the Western psyche through incorporating the five elements of nature as outlined in Dagara cosmology. Finally, in Part Five I offer suggestions for promoting community building in a specifically Western context.

Ka ti sankun koro na gan a tinso
tuon kuti laonta yanmaro.
Ka u ʒin a ti sukie puo
ti yi ka ti nonon ta ti yanon ta.

May those from under our feet
breathe the warmth of community unto us
so that the peace we seek
mounts our bodies and sits on the chairs of our hearts,
sprinkling love and joy around us all.

—PRAYER OF THE AFRICAN MEDICINE MAN

KOUNBATERZIÉ ´DABIRÉ ´GUINIAN

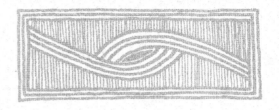

PART ONE

HEALING

IN THE

INDIGENOUS

WORLD

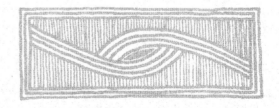

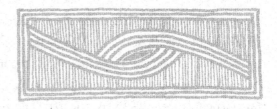

1.

Healing, Ritual, and Community

. . . beneath the skin, beyond the differing features
and into the true heart of being,
fundamentally, we are more alike, my friend,
than we are unalike.
—MAYA ANGELOU

What the indigenous world offers to the modern world centers around the understanding of the concepts of healing, ritual, and community. Indigenous communities have since time immemorial focused their lives and their existence on these issues. *Healing* is central, because it was learned very early that human beings are vulnerable to physiological and biological breakdown, and that this general instability touches all aspects of their existence. They have also learned that the natural environment in which they live is made up of subtle invisible things that, if manipulated in certain ways, can affect the conditions that they intend to heal. *Ritual* is the technology that allows the manipulation of these subtle energies. *Community* is important because there is an understanding that human beings are collectively oriented. The general health and well-being of an individual are connected to a community, and are not something that can be maintained alone or in a vacuum. Healing, ritual, and community—these three elements are vitally linked.

Healing, ritual, and community—the goods that the indigenous world can offer to the West are the very things that the modern world is struggling with. Ritual in the indigenous world is aimed at producing healing, and the loss of such healing in the modern world might be responsible for the loss of community that we see. The problems experienced in the West, from the pain of isolation to the stress of hyperactivity, are brought on by the loss of community.

The problems that come from the loss of ritual are less clear, but it is the absence of ritual that the West is struggling with, the loss of connection with the unseen aspects of the natural world that have the ability to bring the needed healing. The West is also struggling with a confusing notion of ritual, for the word usually refers to some sort of dark, pagan, and archaic practice that has no place in modern society. The only accepted rituals are ceremonial practices with clearly predictable content and outcome, such as what can be seen in the Sunday church service of one of the organized religions. When we talk of ritual here we are talking about something much deeper. We are talking about the weaving of individual persons and gifts into a community that interacts with the forces of the natural world. We are talking about a gathering of people with a clear healing vision and a trusting intent toward the forces of the invisible world.

What villagers bring to a ritual are trust that the invisible forces will heal and the knowledge of what needs healing. These are the only things they know ahead of time; the rest, the shape and outcome of the ritual, is put in the hands of the Great Ones. The road from the felt need for healing to the healing itself is paved with gestures, touch, sound, melody, and cadence, and most of these are spontaneous activities, unpredictable in their outcomes. When villagers act together on their need for healing and engage in such spontaneous gestures, they are requesting the presence of the invisible forces and are participating with those forces in creating a harmony or symbiosis. This partnership replenishes each person by restoring his or her relationship to nature, for among indigenous people the natural world and the Spirit World are closely related, as we will see. Ritual is an art, an art that weaves and dances with symbols, and helping to create that art rejuvenates participants. Everyone comes away from a ritual feeling deeply transformed. This restoration is the healing that ritual is meant to provide.

Indigenous people see the physical world as a reflection of a more complex, subtler, and more lasting yet invisible entity called energy. It is as if we are the shadows of a vibrant and endlessly resourceful intelligence dynamically involved in a process of continuous self-creation. Nothing happens here that did not begin in that unseen world. If something in the physical world is experiencing instability, it is because its energetic correspondent has been experiencing instability. The indigenous understanding is that the material and physical problems that a person encounters are important only because they are an energetic message sent to this visible world. Therefore, people go to that unseen energetic place to try to repair whatever damage or disturbances are being done there, knowing that if things are healed there, things will be healed here. Ritual is the principal tool used to approach that unseen world in a way that will rearrange the structure of the physical world and bring about material transformation.

That we connect with unseen realities, the realities made visible in our symbols, is crucial to the well-being of our psyches. A person who walks through a ritual and ends up feeling charged and invigorated is a blessed recipient of healing waves of energy that no one can see but everyone can benefit from. The full heart of a person blessed in this manner overflows into the needy souls of others, igniting the healing fire most wanted for

self-replenishment. Ritual is central to village life, for it provides the focus and energy that holds the community together, and it provides the
kind of healing that the community most needs to survive.

HUNGER FOR SPIRIT

The West is hungry for Spirit, for the contact with unseen forces that
brings healing. The West's hunger for Spirit, however, comes with cultural constraints. People want to experience the Spirit, the Other World,
but they want to experience it on their own terms. People are quick to mis-
understand or reject teachings that offer them a world they don't recognize.

The first time I introduced a ritual to people in this country, I was at
once brought face-to-face with this fact. It was a sunny summer afternoon
in a natural setting amid impressive redwood trees. It was a men's retreat,
and I had chosen to lead the hundred or so men gathered there in a ritual
of grieving, the sacred shedding of tears to heal the wounds of human
losses. But as soon as I began to speak, I realized these men had no idea
why crying was important. As I struggled to make sense of grief, I realized that I was trying to make familiar a concept that is perhaps more remote to modern people, especially males, than I can imagine. I heard
myself clumsily argue that to shed tears is to release an energy that otherwise will poison the self. "How do you know that?" retaliated an angry
voice inside of me—what I imagined the audience members were saying.
I felt deeply embarrassed, for I was sure that my audience was full of experts who had investigated this field long before. Their faces showed none
of the enthusiasm that communicates understanding.

I finally decided that I needed at least to justify why indigenous people
do ritual grieving, even if I failed to make it apply to modern people. So I
spoke about grief as a cleansing practice that purifies the psyche just as a
bath purifies the body. I stated the danger of unexpressed grief, quoting
an elder who once said that a man who can't cry is a social time bomb. To

my surprise, light began to dawn on the faces of these men as they came to accept the idea of addressing the immense grief buried in their psyches. They understood that they lived in a culture where the expression of grief is almost taboo.

But actually performing a ritual expressing grief proved even harder for these men than accepting the idea of it. They showed tremendous resistance to taking action and preferred to continue talking about the ritual instead of actually entering into it. To express their grief required them to move out of familiar psychological territory to a place where their sense of control faded away—a place where their vulnerability would emerge with all its terrifying effects.

That afternoon we gathered to clean up a spot among the trees and to turn it into a ritual space. Working together was invigorating. It was as if the invisible world participated in its own subtle ways, for among the men there was complete cooperation in preparing the ritual space. I sent them out to find each an object among the trees that represented the loss they needed to grieve. This much they did without resistance.

By then it was dark. The setting of the sun awoke the beings of the night. People's tension rose, as if they felt that these beings saw what was going on and had decided to join in. As we gathered one last time to clear the air before moving on to the ritual proper, various complaints arose. One person expressed his fear of getting into something that might violate his religious beliefs. Another said he was afraid of losing control and therefore leaving the ritual feeling worse than before. These reservations struck a chord with others, who agreed that they thought they had come here to be supported in a safe environment to do safe things.

I felt helpless. On the one hand I could clearly see that the hunger for ritual was being checked against the prescription of social conditioning. On the other hand, I could not understand why they would want to travel so long together, only to turn back within sight of the destination. I tried my best to calm the terrified and to comfort the confused. I agreed with them that true Spirit is a frightening thing to embrace. But I objected to their need for safety. It became a subject of debate.

At last one man quoted someone as saying that healing involves taking a risk with the backing of Spirit. I realized, with relief, that I had sup-
porters in the group. My helplessness disappeared as I exhorted the group
to have faith in Spirit. The group decided to go forward with the ritual.
For four hours tearful voices rose above chants of lament, held together
by the regular beat of a drum. These cries—some of them aimed high as
though seeking to awake a sleeping god or goddess—were loud enough
to bend the tops of many trees, who seemed to echo their sorrow amid the
windy darkness. I thought to myself, the darkness has made everyone
black; this could be anywhere in Africa. Each hour brought the ritual to its
next level of intensity. As people grieved louder, the lament song rose
proportionally with the drum. Everything grieved in unison. The Spirit
lived among us.

In the morning we gathered in a room away from the ritual place to
share what it felt like to be in a ritual space with others, and particularly
how the experience of grieving felt. For most people it was one of the
most highly rewarding things they had ever done. They were still surprised at how deeply they had entered into it and were amazed at the
amount of grief they had released. True, there were a few who could not
get into it, but even they were amazed by what they witnessed in others,
to the point that they regretted not being able to grieve. As I listened carefully to each person's comments, I realized how open the room felt by
contrast to the tension of the day before. People joked with one another.
There was a great deal of humor in the room. They thanked one another
for the mutual support and expressed gratitude for the opportunity of taking part in something so powerful. It was obvious that the group had embraced Spirit.

HEALING, IDENTITY, AND COMMUNITY

What was it that urged these people to search for healing? My sense is that
the West's need for healing is rooted in crises of personal identity and

purpose. Whether they are raised in indigenous or modern culture, there are two things that people crave: the full realization of their innate gifts, and to have these gifts approved, acknowledged, and confirmed. There are countless people in the West whose efforts are sadly wasted because they have no means of expressing their unique genius. In the psyches of such people there is an inner power and authority that fails to shine because the world around them is blind to it.

This implies that our own inner authority needs the fuel of external recognition to inspire us to fulfill our life's purpose, and until this happens, we wait in paralysis for the redemptive social response that rescues us from the dungeon of anonymity. Our own confirmation or acknowledgment of ourselves is not enough. The need to be acknowledged by the society is so primal that if it does not happen in the village, town, or neighborhood, people will go out searching for it. For many people, the support offered by indigenous ritual satiates the soul by providing it with a sense of connection with a greater dimension.

A crisis of identity and purpose is an inner burning that is rarely extinguished by a visit to a career-planning office, by graduation from a prestigious school, or even by years in a successful career. It is a hollowness, a void that threatens to erase meaning in everything people do. This hollowness is reflected in the attraction of indigenous rituals for many Westerners. A romantic approach to the indigenous world has compelled some seekers to feel profoundly ill at ease about not having experienced a ritual initiation, as their counterparts in the indigenous world have experienced.

It is perhaps important to point out that these Westerners may underestimate the depth of their own learning and life experience. Many people would agree that living in the West has its own dangers, which are similar to the dangers to which African youth are exposed during the rituals of initiation. Westerners meet up with tragedy, with powers beyond their control, with challenges that present opportunities for growth and transformation. And these challenges must be recognized as initiatory, even though this initiation is disorganized, unpredictable, and informal, unlike the carefully orchestrated initiatiatory challenges presented to indigenous people. Westerners, like their indigenous counterparts, experience initiation in some form and in a constant manner throughout their life. A person who gets fired at the job faces a life-transforming challenge that must be considered initiatory. A couple facing crisis in their relationship, such as separation or divorce, is on an initiatory path. Initiation is simply a set of challenges presented to an individual so that he or she may grow. Consequently, the troubles we encounter in our paths in the modern world are, in essence, initiatory to the extent that each one of them is life changing.

What is lacking in this rich life experience is a community that observes the individual's growth and certifies that one has passed through an initiatory process. This would not be the kind of certification that gives a person a title in order to pursue a career, but the mere act of seeing and responding, which enables a person, in powerful periods of growth, to behold voices within confirmed by voices from the community without. The issue for Westerners is not so much the absence of initiation as it is the absence of a community to recognize initiatory passages. Tribal life is full of public ritual initiations marking the various stages of a person's life. From the rituals of birth to the funeral rituals at death, every person's life journey is clearly highlighted with the milestones of transformational rituals. To the extent that these rituals are challenging and involve hardship, they are comparable to the challenges life presents to individuals in the Western world.

Though we will look further into the dynamics of community later on in this book, I would like to stress at this point that where mentors and elders are lacking, and where initiation in one form or another is not recognized, there can be no support system capable of curbing the intense sense of aloneness that haunts the psyche of the modern person. Only being part of a community will address the loneliness of modern people.

But I have learned that there is in many Western people a strong resistance to joining community because of all the flaws apparent in the intentional communities they have seen. Part of this resistance stems perhaps from a disappointed idealism, a demand that a community be perfect. But in fact an intentional community in the West is a place where people agree to work at becoming better connected to one another. Even indigenous communities, which we often praise, are far from being perfect. They certainly offer a great deal in the area of maintaining connection both with other people and with Spirit and the Other World. But in their pursuit of the Spirit, they may have forgotten to integrate it with matter, hence their deprivation in terms of the basic material necessities of life.

People's resistance to community in the West may also come from an undeveloped sense of personhood. Someone who believes that community exists in order to provide for his or her needs without having to give anything in response will probably never find the right community. In this case resistance arises because of old, unmet psychological needs. Since giving is the modus operandi of community, proper spiritual and emotional clarity within are necessary for establishing a sense of belonging. Otherwise, people will tend to look for Spirit using the same compulsive methods they use to search for material goods.

SPIRIT AND HEALING

Because healing in the indigenous world includes the dimension of Spirit, definitions of illness extend also to the unseen worlds of mind and Spirit. When my younger brother first went off to college in Ouagadougou, he had tremendous problems comprehending his course work. He understood immediately that he was ill, and that the tribal shamans rather than teachers could help him, so he returned to the village for a consultation. How did he know he was ill? Because the inability to perceive, the inability to understand, to indigenous people is symptomatic of an illness. If your psyche is disordered or deficient or overcharged, blocks are created in you that prevent comprehension and remembering. To open up the channels in you so that whatever energy you need can flow freely is not the task of the teacher; it is the task of the shaman. The shaman, who may not know anything about reading or writing or mathematics or physics, will have a way of fine-tuning a student's brain and energetic configuration so that he or she can absorb the material.

Another form of this illness is the inability to accept or even tolerate those who are different from us. Worse, this inability encourages suspicion, fear, and resentment. Thus it is an illness of the collective psyche when different cultures don't understand one another. The history of humankind is plagued by this psychic disease that has caused much pain and disappointment in the world.

Methods of healing must take into account the energetic or spiritual condition that is in turmoil, thereby affecting the physical condition. If you focus only on the physical translation of the underlying energetic disorder, then you are ignoring the source of the physical illness. If you address only the physical problem, then you end up perhaps with a cure, which fixes the physical condition, providing a momentary sense of victory over debilitation. But this act denies the needs of the energy, the adjustment of Spirit needed to make the cure last. Sooner or later this disordered energy will figure out a new way to affect the physical body, often in a new and more virulent manner than it did originally. If you instead address the energy of the mind and Spirit, whose status is affecting the physical body, then you are likely to heal truly. Hence, in the wisdom of indigenous concepts of healing, all healing must begin by first addressing the energetic problems, and ritual is the crucible where this transformation and healing occur.

HEALING AND AWARENESS

Ritual is aimed at increasing our awareness, for awareness of the existence of the reality beyond the palpable world that we live in is one of the keys to transforming an individual. Ritual can shake a person free from the rigidity of that part of the ego that wants to limit growth and experience. The geography of human consciousness is very expansive, almost without limit. A shaman in my village once told me, "Our minds know better than we are able and willing to admit, and we are witness to many more things than we are willing to accept. The spirit and the mind are one. Their vision is greater, much greater than the vision we experience in the ordinary world." If something comes into our lives and we deny it by labeling it impossible, an indigenous elder would interpret this way of thinking as a manifestation of our own rigidity in the face of new possibilities. In the mind of a villager, the unreal is just a new and yet-unconfirmed reality in the vocabulary of consciousness. It is brought to us by the ancestors. A little hospitality toward it will suffice to make it part of us. In short, the indigenous mind does not admit impossibility. It defines itself by not rejecting the unfamiliar, and it therefore thrives on mysteries and magic. Such a mind gives ample space to the invisible because the invisible holds the key to the wisdom of the universe.

Eventually such awareness becomes an honoring of the shadowy and hidden parts of ourselves, those parts of ourselves that are invisible. There is such a thing as a spirit person and a physical person, and more often than not the physical being is so detached from the spirit that one feels split inside. Awareness should ultimately lead to an attempt to bring these two parts of the person together to become one.

A physical body alone cannot have any sort of direction in this life, so it is important to recognize that the body is an extension of the spirit, and the spirit is an extension of the body, and that the two are inseparable, with a communication that goes both ways. This is nothing supernatural, it is just what it is. It is as though we are adrift in space during our life, and like an astronaut circling the earth we too need to keep in touch with a base that will tell us how to navigate and maneuver. Our base is in the Spirit World, and ritual helps us open our channel again to that world. This is why the indigenous mind sees Spirit or the potential for the existence of Spirit in every object; we are hungry for instructions in navigating an often-uncertain world.

RITUAL, MEMORY, AND PURPOSE

Ritual provides not only healing but also the recovery of memory and the reaffirmation of each individual's life purpose. How does ritual recover memory? When we focus our attention on the energetic aspects of individuals and of nature that animate and motivate us, we become aware of images and emotional impressions that are unusual, extremely compelling, and as a result, captivating in terms of the amount of attention they demand. Inside ritual and sacred space where energies are being woven, people's imagination and consciousness can be moved through time backward or forward. It is as if the awakened psyche is pulled toward those materials it was not able to recall otherwise. This is a shamanic journey, and it can be a very useful tool for entering these depths of time and space without actually having to expand energy and move physically. The kind of memory that we are talking about here is something very personal, very compelling, and very transforming.

I remember one example of a white man who was involved in an African-style ritual in England who was asked to play a *djembe* during the ritual. He played the drum nonstop for nearly ten hours. Later on he said that after a few hours, he found himself in an African village drumming with a community of villagers, and the energy was so strong that he didn't realize that time was flowing. How can you explain this other than to say that the ritual invoked something that allowed this person to dive into a place of memory where he remembered why he was so good at drumming? In other words, he had done it before. This is not an idea new in the history of Western thought. For instance, Aristotle, in his logical discourses, posits that a mathematician can ultimately understand mathematics only if it is originally in his nature to do so, if there is some memory present initially upon which all later training and education can build. In the understanding of most indigenous people, learning of all sorts is nothing more than remembering what you already know.

One's purpose, which among indigenous people is found through remembering, is linked to both the physical world and to the Spirit World. We look to the Spirit World for the ultimate helper who assists the individual in fulfilling her or his purpose. This spirit is seen as something like a guardian angel would be seen in the West, and we call this spirit the Siura. We look to the physical world, the community of people, for help in remembering our purpose. Purpose is not something that is assigned to a person by his or her community. Purpose is something that the individual has framed and articulated *prior to* coming into a community. This purpose is known to the village even before the individual's birth.

In our village everyone gets excited when they hear a woman has become pregnant. Everyone asks, "Why is this person being sent to us at this time? What gifts will this person have that our community needs?" A special ritual is held to answer these questions. Expert shamans gather with the mother of the fetus and place her under hypnosis. They contact the life force behind the fetus and ask it to speak using the mother's voice. The shamans then converse with the fetus, asking it why it is coming into the world and what work it intends to do. The fetus responds in ways that suggest that the individual has first presented a proposal for his or her life purpose to some council of elders in the Spirit World. Once the council approves the proposal, it gives the individual permission to be born into a physical body. In this way the community of people welcoming an infant has some idea of that individual's intentions for life, and it is then the responsibility of that community to help the person continue to remember and focus on her or his chosen life purpose.

If the ritual and sacred method of divining purpose are not available, an individual's purpose can still be identified by noting what the individual is naturally drawn to. Certain things, like art or construction or design or storytelling, will trigger some excitement in the person. This feeling is the key to identifying one's purpose. Therefore it is not necessary for people in the modern world to go to some kind of wise man or authority to have their purpose assigned to them. The leadership that they need lies within their own relationship to the world of Spirit and the ancestors. Your purpose is linked to, and monitored by, the spirits in the unseen world. The unseen world, the world of the ancestral spirits, has authorized your purpose, giving you the right to possess the physical body and consciousness needed to exist in this material world.

Your Siura is behind you, trying to work with you as closely as possible to keep you on the path of your purpose, speaking to you through your inspiration, your dreams, and your instincts. An offering to your Siura now and then at an ancestor altar or any altar is appropriate, a token of appreciation for the diligence and leadership they have shown toward your purpose.

Purpose begins with the individual, and the sum total of all the individuals' purposes creates the community's purpose. The community thus takes upon itself the responsibility of nurturing and protecting the individual, because the individual, knowing her or his purpose, will then invest energy in sustaining the community. There is a certain reciprocity at work here, because the community recognizes that its own vitality is based in the support and protection of each of its individuals, especially in the constant support and reminding of each individual of his or her purpose. The individual, knowing this, in turn delivers to the community the gifts that the community has successfully awakened in him or her.

The presence of a community to awaken our gifts in us is necessary because the process of being born tends to erase our memory of why we came here. And the blindness that we have toward our purpose is progressive. Early in life you are still at that place where you feel that you might do something. Children's vitality and enthusiasm are reminiscent of the forces that motivated them to come here. Of course, the coldness of this world and the rather clear hostility that most of us encounter trying to survive discourage us from the kind of purpose that we were originally so enthused about. Even within the indigenous context, there is a need for ritual to make sure that the damage done to you by society, to the point where your enthusiasm is tampered with, is repaired, so that you can embrace your purpose fully. Being born into this world is a trying experience. Whatever enthusiasm you bring with you here can be toned down and radically edited simply as a result of being here. The time of physiological transformation when you are growing up is particularly trying, and in this process a toll is taken on your sense of purpose, including forgetting. All of these changes at the time of puberty have a deep influence on the dynamics of relationship, both with the unseen world and the world that can be seen.

Also, for most young people, the stark visibility of the seen world affects their perception of the unseen world. Discrimination begins when you say that you can touch this and that, and therefore the reality of the tangible begins to supersede the reality of the intangible. If you are not exposed to community ritual, you are vulnerable to growing away from Spirit, until you die. The physiological signs of puberty mark a time when a specific type of ritual is called for, one designed to reconnect the person with the world of the spirits and their purpose, and this is what we call initiation. Later in the book we will speak more of rituals of initiation, but for now what is important is that rituals of all kinds help to reawaken the intensity that brought us here. Making ritual a part of daily life will help to rekindle the intensity that keeps us on the path of our purpose.

In the later chapters of this book, where we discuss how to conduct rituals, many details about what must be done in the ritual are not included. Ritual is by its nature a communal activity and an act of creation. The people involved must develop these details themselves to fit the particular need that is being addressed. The ritual must create a certain kind of energy that can embrace the individuals involved, allowing them to expand their awareness and undergo the transformation necessary to become healed. Ritual is not a rigid thing. Simply by virtue of being a human being, one is an authority on creating ritual.

If people know the problem that they are confronting, they are capable of devising a ritual that will handle this problem. A recipe that someone brings from somewhere else will not solve the problem. If you start by trusting yourself and your ability to address an issue symbolically, you are likely to deepen your experience in designing ritual. There are no cookbooks, and there is no need for some master to be staring over your shoulder when a ritual is designed. Rituals never like to be done the same way twice, for they would rather reflect the versatility of human imagination than its corresponding power to create stagnation and rigidity. Simply take into account the geography you are in, your place in time, the nature of the problem, and the nature of the community of people and spirits that have been called for the ritual, and you will end up with something that is very transforming. Ritual is a tribute to the human capacity to create, remember, and imagine, and to apply that imagination for the benefit of the community. One of the greatest barriers to memory and imagination is the lack of self-trust, for if you don't trust yourself to be involved in transforming that which needs to be changed, then you end up waiting for someone else to come along and do the work for you. This leads to a constant state of dependence on some external authority, when the means to achieving what you want sits within yourself.

Ritual, community, and healing—these three are so intertwined in the indigenous world that to speak of one of them is to speak of them all. *Ritual*, communally designed, helps the individual remember his or her purpose, and such remembering brings healing both to the individual and the community. The *community* exists, in part, to safeguard the purpose of each person within it and to awaken the memory of that purpose by recognizing the unique gifts each individual brings to this world. *Healing* comes when the individual remembers his or her identity—the purpose chosen in the world of ancestral wisdom—and reconnects with that world of Spirit. Human beings long for connection, and our sense of usefulness derives from the feeling of connectedness. When we are connected—to our own purpose, to the community around us, and to our spiritual wisdom—we are able to live and act with authentic effectiveness.

In order for ritual to manifest its full power, it must be connected to the world of nature, and to this topic we now turn. To attend to the world of Spirit, for indigenous people, is to attend to the geography in which you find yourself. We must try, therefore, to understand the indigenous experiences of nature.

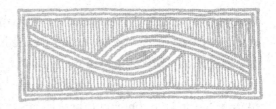

2.

The Healing Power
of Nature

When I was a child, I spoke like a child,
I thought like a child, I reasoned like a child;
when I became a man, I gave up childish ways.
For now we see as in a darkened mirror,
but then face-to-face.
Now I know in part; then I shall understand fully,
even as I have been fully understood.

—1 CORINTHIANS 13

Nature is the foundation of indigenous life. Without nature, concepts of community, purpose, and healing would be meaningless. The idea of a person born with a purpose, a purpose that needs to be supported by an active community presence, and the idea of working with subtle energies for balance and healing would be only grandiose notions in the absence of nature as the playground, as the school where the children can play and study. Our relationship to the natural world and its natural laws determines whether or not we are healed. Nature, therefore, is the foundation of healing, and the type of nature that surrounds a community at the time of doing a ritual determines the types of ritual that are appropriate and the content of these rituals. We are talking about a way of dealing with an energetic world and energetic issues that borrows from what already exists, not what has been invented, manufactured, or created by humans to satisfy some material purpose. In other words, every tree, plant, hill, mountain, rock, and each thing that was here before us emanates or vibrates at a subtle energy that has healing power whether we know it or not. So if something in us must change, spending time in nature provides a good beginning. This means that within nature, within the natural world, are all of the materials and tenets needed for healing human beings. Nature is the textbook for those who care to study it and the storehouse of remedies for human ills.

The natural world is an integral part of an indigenous community. Village people envision the community as including the geography and the natural world that surrounds and contains the people. The close relationship between people and place is symbolized by the bond that indigenous people recognize between a person and his or her place of birth, and also in the fact that any ritual that is performed is viewed as being tied to the geography where it takes place. The theory behind this close connection between geography and people is that different parts of the earth are tied to specific forces in the Other World, just as different parts of the human body are linked to specific function. People will thus have a special relationship with the forces in the Other World that correspond to their birthplace. In other words, we are more or less the function of that part of the earth we are born into. To interact properly with another part of the earth requires the "approval" of our original earth. Hence some people believe that we choose not only our parents but also our place of birth.

This is simply another way of emphasizing the importance of nature, for geography and nature are not really dissimilar. Being born into this world in a particular place is like having the signature of that place stamped upon you. The essence of your place of birth cloaks and protects your walk through this life, and whatever you do becomes registered in the ledger of that geography. You can end up thousands of miles away from your birthplace, and if you are involved in a healing ritual that is meant to work, you have to invoke the spirits that are at the place where you were born in addition to those who are natives of the place you are in. The spirits that witnessed your birth at that place are still there, and your calling them will awaken their attention in your direction. If you embrace this concept, you will find that human mobility does not remove a person's original connection to the birthplace. Your footprints still lead back to the place where you began. Any time there is a thought or memory of the origin, or an allusion to the origin, or more specifically a prayer that addresses your roots and the nature of your origin, then vast forces in the universe are unleashed. It does not matter whether you feel good about your past or not. It matters only that you feel. The feeling is a sign that you still respond to these forces of the origin. In fact, feeling bad about one's origin is a sign that the forces in it want a healing between you and them.

It is useful to remember the subtle things that one was aware of as a small child. The memory of being tucked into bed at night by your parents, who turned the light off as they left your room, followed by the appearance of a loving being who nourished your imagination just as fairy tales do cannot and should not be forgotten. Most of us will realize that we had a relationship with the parallel reality that surrounded us in the geography where we were born, a reality that could both contradict what we observed among the adults who surrounded us, as well as attract our attention more than the one the adults were trying to instruct us to become aware of. This remembrance of the parallel world of our childhood is the place we can go to reestablish our connection with the natural world, the connection between us and the geography of our birthplace.

MEETING A BEING FROM THE OTHER WORLD

I have told earlier, in *Of Water and the Spirit*, my own rather dramatic experience as a small child in nature. The vivid memory of a childhood experience that still follows me is connected with an experience in nature with a rabbit. I remember that day when my mother took me along to fetch wood. It is not uncommon to see women with a baby on the back tightly tied going into the bush to gather wood for cooking. My mother tied me that way one of those days when she was going to the bush, and of course, because of my liking for nature, when we got there she laid me down and I just took off. The immediate habit was to go looking for live things, and I would run after anything that was alive and try to catch it. It so happened that in running from one bush to another, I came upon a rabbit, and that was a big thing for a child. I could feel my heartbeat increasing and my adrenaline shooting, because I knew that it would be great if I could catch this little thing. I wanted a really good hunting experience, and when the rabbit disappeared inside a bush, that increased my hunting instincts, for I knew that the rabbit was taking refuge in there. I decided not to run, and I started walking slowly so as not to scare it. The bush was made of lumps of grass, what you may call ferns, and I knew that the rabbit was going to be hiding in one of these. I pulled open one and there was nothing there, I pulled open another and there was nothing there, and then there was only one left.

I moved the last clump of grass, and I wasn't prepared for what I saw. Instead of the rabbit, there was something extraordinary, like a doll, a doll about a foot tall of a human being, except that the doll was alive, sitting on something like a tiny chair. But I wasn't interested in the chair, I was interested in the location where it was sitting. It was above something more like a window, as though you were looking through a window seeing the sky of an immense world, except that the sky was below. But the little man wasn't falling through this window, he was just sitting there. I had been making a gesture to leap with all of my weight onto the rabbit, knowing that if I fell on it I would suffocate it, but this gesture stopped halfway down. I was frozen by the sight that appeared in front of me. Worse, the little being began to speak, telling me in a thin voice, "I have been watching you for a long time, ever since your mother started bringing you here. Why do you want to hurt the rabbit, your little brother? What did he do to you, little one? Be friendly to him from now on. He too likes the fresh air of this place, he too has a mother who cares for him. What would his mother say if you hurt him? Now go because your own mother is worried."

At the time, it made no sense to hear this. What was captivating to me was the fact that I was dealing with a person smaller than me, yet older than me, with a long white beard, sitting in the wrong place at the wrong time, talking to me. Too many pieces of information, each requiring very careful attention, were coming into me, and I couldn't deal with all of them at once. All I could notice was that the rabbit was still there, but it was behind this mysterious halolike window. To me the view through the window looked like the sky, like the blue sky, and in it was something that looked like a cloud, but it was not a cloud. Nothing was quite like what we normally see. Everything looked as if it could be this or that, but there was always something missing to make it totally right.

The truth of it is that I never made sense of what happened. All I remembered is that after the little man spoke I heard the sound of my name being called: "Malidoma, please answer me! Where are you?" It was a familiar voice, the voice of my mother. When I finally reconnected with her, it was late during the day, but we had arrived there in the early part of the day, about midmorning. I found myself wondering what had happened in that short period of time, which had encompassed an entire day. My mother was breathless, as if she had been looking for me with much trepidation for the whole day. I felt quite fine, and when I told her that I was running after a rabbit and I saw an old man and he told me that I shouldn't hurt rabbits she became panicked. I couldn't understand why my mother wasn't as calm as I was, for I felt as though I'd only been gone for five minutes, and she was acting as though I'd been gone for the whole day.

When I said that I'd seen the old man she screamed that I'd seen a *kontomblé* (which is the Dagara word for beings from the Other Side of reality, the world of Spirit). I could not remember having heard about these little beings before. This was good because I knew I would not have reacted the way I did. All I knew was that I had seen a tiny man who was very old, and he told me not to hurt rabbits. This was indeed my first serious connection with nature and the magic in it. This experience allowed me later on to wonder what other things might be hiding out there in nature that we choose not to notice, or that we are not open enough to allow into the view of our consciousness. Had I not encountered beings like them many more times as an educated adult and conversed with them while taping their voices with their permission for my own record, I think I would have dismissed my original experience as a kind of hallucination. Even now, I still have one reservation about them: it is the fact that they are not willing to show me everything about themselves, on the grounds that it will endanger me. They think that certain mental conditionings—they wouldn't say which ones—that I have contracted abroad have weakened my psyche's ability to embrace the broader spectrum of reality that their world offers without severely impairing my sense of this world's reality.

In Africa in general, and particularly in that region of Africa, no one is surprised when you talk about these beings, because everybody knows about the little beings that are very intelligent and very powerful who live in a dimension that is very close to our dimension. I have, however, never again encountered them exactly the way that I did when I was so young. My enduring reaction to this experience tells me that a lot more things exist in nature than that which our own sight is able to grasp, and these things can shape very strongly the way we see reality around us. Maybe we would become candidates for some serious magic if we could enter nature with a little more curiosity, a little more openness, and even with a sense of a quest, a quest to commune with and to be with a realm that is far more sophisticated than its physical ruggedness reveals.

I still ask why that *kontomblé* chose to appear to me at that very time, at that very age. I can draw from this that the spirit of a little child radiates something that can easily interact with the energies of nature. It may very well be that my experience with pursuing that rabbit intensified something in me that led to the opening of that very space. That encounter has made me very aware of the existence of something behind the veil of nature that very likely keeps an eye on every human being. It has made me wonder, every time I am walking in nature, about who is looking at me, who is observing me, and how many eyes are seeing everything that I do without my knowing it. It has made me want to interact with these intelligences, with these beings that are so capable of noticing our human actions. I have always been curious about what would happen if we were to go out into nature and find ourselves being welcomed by some *kontomblé* elf who shows up to us saying, "Thanks for coming into our world. Let me show you around." What would we do to nature from then on if we knew that in order for these encounters to occur, nature requires that it be kept the way it is?

COMMUNION WITH NATURE

When I was twenty, I experienced another profound and moving interaction with nature, this time as part of the rituals of initiation with other villagers. The story of the green lady appeared in *Of Water and the Spirit* as a part of the larger story of my traditional initiation, but it stands alone well, worth pairing with the rabbit story.

When I first returned home to the village after leaving the missionary school, I felt a sense of nostalgia that seemed as though it would never be satisfied. My fifteen years in Western institutions had created a huge gap between me and my people. Returning home was not satisfactory, because I felt that I didn't belong. I returned to my village not being able to speak in the language of my people and not being able to embrace their manners, because I found the customs disgusting.

To help me reintegrate into my family and village, the elders decided that I should undergo the initiation rituals appropriate to the boys of the village who are on the verge of puberty. There I was, taking part in processes with boys many years younger than I. The pressure on me not to fail was enormous, for failing initiation rituals could have meant death (for some of the rituals are physically dangerous) or the inability to reconnect with my people and be accepted as an adult.

The initiation processes were physically excruciating. On this particular afternoon, I had exhausted every resource in trying to outwit the elders who had given me the assignment to sit down and look at a tree until its true nature was revealed. The idea, of course, was completely absurd, because my rather Westernized mind (I had by that time been educated for fifteen years in French mission schools) was totally unable to grasp what it meant just to sit down and look at a tree. The experience was made worse by complete physical discomfort. I remember well the temperature of a hundred and ten degrees, my nakedness, sweat, and hunger, the hot gravel and crawling ants. In the middle of all of this I was being asked to ignore the discomfort and focus my attention on a tree—a stupid exercise, I thought. After about thirty hours of this excruciating discomfort, including the shame of being caught trying to lie about what I was experiencing in order to fool the elders into thinking I had "gotten it," I realized that the one thing I had to do was to find some way to end the ordeal. I had moved to a critical juncture: I could give up and terminate the exercise right there, which would mean terminating my initiation. Or I could find some way through.

I felt shame and failure, and I was crying. What was wrong with me that I could not do what I was asked to do? I was failing at an initiation task, and my sense of ostracism from my peers—they hadn't been taken away from home and asked to endure fifteen years in a foreign culture— became even more painful and intolerable. Through my tears, however, I continued to keep an eye on the tree. As I looked at it, I suddenly began speaking to it, as if I had finally discovered that it had a life of its own. I told it all about my discontent and my sadness and how I felt that it had abandoned me to the shame of lying and of being laughed at.

I then spoke to the tree again, not angrily, but respectfully. I told her that, after all, it was not her fault that I could not see, but mine. I simply lacked the ability. What I really needed to do was to come to terms with my own emptiness and lack of sight, because I knew *she* would always be there when I needed to use her to take a good look at my own shortcomings and inadequacies.

What happened next is the kind of experience that, like the encounter with the rabbit, molded my perception forever. The tree that I had been watching for so long was no longer there, and in its place was a beautiful green lady. I do not know if the tree became her, or if she stepped out of the tree, but this really doesn't matter. Where the tree had been there was now a figure that looked like a human being, in the shape of a woman, very tall, probably seven and a half feet tall. Her tunic was silky and black, and she wore a veil over her face, and when I looked again, she had lifted the veil, revealing an unearthly face. I call her the green lady because she was green, her skin was green. But the greenness in her had nothing to do with the color of her skin. She was green from the inside out, as if her body were filled with green fluid. I do not know how I knew this, but this green was the expression of immeasurable love.

What I felt was of an intensity similar to what I had experienced with the rabbit and the little *kontomblé*. As soon as she appeared I felt some sort of shock that enveloped my whole body. It produced in me a feeling of the type that I had never experienced before and that I've never experienced again. There was a magnetic pull toward her, and I don't know how I got there, whether I crawled or ran, but I found myself in her arms. It was a homecoming of utmost healing. I was sobbing as I had never done before, for I felt that I was in the hands of the ultimate divine being, hands that provided the ultimate sense of acceptance and home that could never be denied.

I had no idea how long I was in her arms, but it felt like a long time. I had no intention of ending this embrace. Having finally gotten this feeling, this support, this love, I had the feeling that all we needed to do was just go home and live happily ever after. But then I realized that she was telling me that she needed to go, and I needed to go too. Of course, that was not part of my plan, and as a result I found myself clinging to her. How could she go without me? I was with her, holding her totally in my hands, so I held her more strongly. It was then that a strange thing happened, which I have never been able to figure out, changing the softness of her feminine body into some kind of ruggedness that became more and more uncomfortable. With a pleading gesture I lifted my head to beg her to stay, and my eyes told me that I was hugging the tree. The feeling was very humbling. I felt at first that I had been deceived, yet my body and spirit felt very subdued, with an almost religious posture. I didn't dwell in the feeling of being tricked, because the strong feeling of the reality of what I had experienced was still present. I was bitterly disappointed at not being able to go with her, and disappointed that such a powerful and loving being had been turned back into a tree. As I sobbed holding the tree, I became aware of the comments that the elders who had been watching me were making. I heard one of them say, "They are always like this. First, they resist and play dumb when there are a lot of things waiting to be done, and then when it happens, they won't let it go, either. Children are so full of contradictions. The very experience you rejected before with lies, you are now accepting without apology."

This last sentence seemed to have been directed at me. I looked up at the elder who spoke. He met my eyes, and I felt no further need to be holding on to the tree. Hours had passed, and the sun had already set. "Go find something to eat, and make your bed for the night," he said gently.

What can one make of my experience? It could easily be dismissed on the grounds of some well-known theories. After all wasn't it very hot that day? What kinds of hallucinations might arise in a person who is dehydrated, hot, and hungry? I've followed that line of reasoning myself many times, only to turn back from it ultimately. Two things have brought me back from doubt. The first is my continued interaction, as a Western-educated adult, with the Other World, particularly the *kontomblé*. The other thing is that elders who were there with me that day were obviously sharing my experience. These witnesses had seen what I had seen, and they were not dehydrated or thirsty. This tells me that more things exist than what my powerful Western education can explain. And for some reason, the things I cannot explain using my Western education seem much more interesting to me than the mundane facts of everyday experience. Hence my deliberate attempt to share these experiences.

My experience with the green lady raises an important issue, namely, the true identity of the elements of nature. What if they are not inanimate objects, as people in the West have been taught to believe, but rather living presences? How would we need to change if we granted to a tree the kind of life that we usually reserve for so-called intelligent beings? If you peek long enough into the natural world—the trees, the hills, the rivers, and all natural things—you start to realize that their spirit is much bigger than what can be seen, that the visible part of nature is only a small portion of what nature is. The elders say that there is much, much more to seeing than simple sight. To me at least, the green lady is a being who took that form to convince me of the vitality inside that tree.

Nature shows itself in some unique way to every individual during his or her initiation, and I know of the stories of many other people who have been touched in this way by nature. The deepest dimension of my own transformation came about through being touched in this way. My jumpy, doubting mind began to find some rest. The fires in me of alienation, pride, and anger began to be quenched by the waters of accepting love. I no longer felt like a proud, wounded outsider. The experience with the green lady resolved that, for all of a sudden I belonged. I could feel it, I could sense it, I was in it. The isolation brought about by becoming alienated from my own native language and able to speak only in the language of the colonizer was wiped out in one shot with the experience with the green lady. She changed me from deep inside. She allowed me to break through the wall of perception that my Western education had erected in me, and she connected me intimately with nature, the way my fellow villagers experienced it. She had brought me back home.

My intellect cannot logically explain or justify it, but my heart, every time I am brought to remember that experience again, leaps out of me with such force that the objections of my mind are put to rest. I relive the intensity and cannot deny the reality that I experienced. My own experience and the similar experiences of others are undeniable examples of the healing power of nature, not only as deeply transformative but as an experience that can radically widen the horizon of one's perception.

This radical connection to nature that I am speaking of is difficult in the West, where any emotionally powerful experience can be dissected and explained away by the intellect as some example of a personal psychological aberration. I have watched such diminishing in my work with ritual in the West. I have seen situations where people experience something so radical that they are almost frantic in telling about it. Because the others present did not participate in this person's experience, they tell the person to calm down, offering alternative, usually more logical and rational, explanations for the person's experience. I notice that my heart hurts whenever someone begins to dissect in psychological or political terms such a powerful and intimate experience. Such behavior only serves to reinforce the notion, common to the Western mind, that there is a division between the real and the supernatural. And all I can say is that at best this dilemma illustrates the line dividing the modern mind from the indigenous mind, not the line between truth and falsehood.

How can modern society accept that the power and vitality in something so apparently inanimate as a tree could touch us deeply and bring about a transformation so profound as to be healing? How do you open people to the possibility that nature has this sort of power and vitality to offer to them? In order to realize the power in nature, we must bring a willingness to consider that something has had its hand in the design of the natural world. What if the appearance of the natural world is the result of something more than the historical accumulation of random geological and natural phenomena? From my own experience I have found that appreciation of the power of nature is increased by inviting people into a ritual space that is directly linked to nature.

After the experience with the green lady, I couldn't get myself to cut a live tree, because I never knew what I was cutting, what sort of spirit might live in the tree that I would be cutting. Every time I walk in nature, especially among trees, I have this feeling of the presence of spirits watching me, similar to the feeling I had after meeting the *kontomblé* with the rabbit. It is almost as though the trees have eyes that follow me in what I am doing and where I am going, and so I have to humble myself. I cannot but wonder about what is the real nature of trees, if they are not simply a source of lumber. What kind of window to the Other World do they represent? Are they really as immobile as they seem to be? Do they have some vitality aside from their physical form that we need to grapple with? What is it that they are conscious of that we need to connect with?

NATURE AND HOME

The profoundness of my experiences with the *kontomblé* and the green lady, along with many other transforming experiences of nature, have helped me to understand the deep reverence with which indigenous people view nature. They view it as their first home, the home that holds the wisdom of the cosmos. To many Westerners, indigenous people's reluctance to disturb the balance of nature has looked like failure to use the raw materials that are just waiting to be harvested and developed. For indigenous people, by contrast, nature is profoundly intelligent *as it stands*, and human beings would do well to learn from its wisdom. An example from Dagara philosophy illustrates my point.

The Source of all, the Dagara believe, has no word. It has no word because meaning is produced instantly, like a cosmic and timeless awareness.

So to the Dagara, there is an understood hierarchy of consciousness. The elements of nature, especially the trees and plants, are the most intelligent beings because they do not need words to communicate. They live closer to the meaning behind language. The next most intelligent species are the animals, because they use only a minimum of uttered communication, so their language is closer to the Source, the world of intrinsic meaning. The last in the hierarchy is the human species, who must rely on words to communicate—and words are but a remote reflection of meaning, like the shadows on the wall of Plato's cave. Wise men and women in the indigenous world argue that humans are cursed by the language they possess, or that possess them. Language, they insist, is an instrument of distance from meaning, an unfortunate necessity that we can't live without but that is so hard to live with.

For indigenous people, *to utter* means two things: first, it signifies nostalgia for our true home, because language tempts us with the possibility of returning home to meaning. And where does meaning reside in its fullness? In nature. So language implies nostalgia for our true home, which is nature. The word *nostalgia* here should not be taken lightly. It implies that language as we have it is a vehicle toward the Source but should never be mistaken for the Source itself.

Second, *to utter* means to be in exile. Indeed, to the Dagara, every time we speak, it is as though we are confessing our own exile, our distance from the Source. The ability to utter testifies to the fact that we are far removed from the vast array of meaning that is our home. For if we were home, we would not feel the need to journey there. At the Source, words would not be necessary, for meaning would be produced instantly. We could see, feel, and touch the results of someone's thought instead of relying on words to give us a picture of it; thought would instantly produce the thing. This is perhaps the indigenous version of the biblical *"et verbum carum factum est, "* "and the word was made flesh."

But the good news is that using language also means that we are on our way back home, journeying to the source of meaning. Those who can't stand being trapped in a place where language tends to distort move into poetry, chant, rhythm, and ritual to speed up their journey home. Poetry and ritual evoke the world behind words, the world of meaning that resides, in its fullness, in nature.

When I connect these last ideas with the experience I had as a child with the rabbit or in my initiation with the green lady, I become aware of some important questions. Namely, does the comfort we seem to desire in the West, to live in a clean, well-lit place, built with wood and the products of nature, match what we would have had if these pieces of wood had been left in place? Are we perhaps also trying to merge with nature, but by way of a different route? Perhaps there is more than one way to come home to Mother Nature.

But in order to surround ourselves with the products of nature, we have had to remove those products from their original, living form. What is the value in creating another route to nature if by creating it we have effaced an already existing one? If our destiny as human beings—as Spirit experiencing physical form—is to become conscious, to become aware of our place and role in the cosmos, why should we rebuild the road that we are going to travel if such a road already exists? To the pain of defacing nature we would be adding the pain of building a different road back to it.

My experiences with the rabbit and the green lady held for me one fundamental lesson, namely that nature indeed is the doorway to a home. It is the knowledge of this home in nature that has led indigenous people not to strive to make their dwellings comfortable. It is as if once you are aware of the comfort that awaits you out there in the natural world, you have very little interest in creating some other better home. When you are aware of the home you have in nature, then you have a sense of home wherever you are, and that sense of comfort follows you to whatever hut or mud home you have built. Having a real sense of home within you tends to make it unnecessary to upgrade your hut into a carpeted, well-lit place.

NATURE AND COMMUNITY

My experience with the green lady also taught me important lessons about the nature of community and healing. Community is about communion, about serving, about being intimately connected. The intimate connections one has in a community cloak the individual with love and acceptance, making that individual feel extremely at home. Home here does not mean some territorial construction, a mere roof over one's head. It is, rather, the place you belong. My experience with the green lady healed my alienation from my people and from nature, restoring me to the places I most deeply belonged.

All of us carry within ourselves something that is waiting for the right moment when it can burst out and repair the particular separation that we are experiencing. My own experience tells me a lot about exile and nostalgia. How many of us are in a state of exile, waiting for the green lady to bring us home to a place of reconciliation? How many people in the West, supposedly at home, nevertheless experience terrific nostalgia and a strongly felt desire to belong? They know that there is a home somewhere, and if they could find it, they would go to it. I imagine that all of the people who feel this way are people who are being beckoned by the green lady to come home.

The feeling of nostalgia signals that there is indeed a home somewhere; that home knows where we are, but it cannot come here, for we have to go out and meet it. That home needs us just as much as we need it, and it can call to us only by injecting us with some feeling that we experience as nostalgia or even as exile. We could blame society and culture or industrialization or the nature of economics for these feelings, but what still remains is the fact that nature is still alive in us, and that is why we feel we are in exile. The green lady has a way of keeping that nature in us so alive that we cannot rest until we come home. The call to come home to the natural world translates as feeling exiled, feeling alienated, feeling like a maladjusted Westerner, feeling as though you can't fit in the way society wants you to fit in to be recognized as a person. This is what triggers the feelings of hopelessness. The people who feel the most hopeless are probably the ones in whom the green lady's power resonates with greatest intensity, because the stronger she calls, the more alienated and desperate you will feel. The green lady emerging from a tree resolved the issues of my own homecoming. Whenever I encounter someone who feels alienated, who feels not at home, I realize that person could use a little bit of the green lady's experience.

A community is held together by emotional ties that result in a conscious feeling of connection, and this feeling of connection is the essence of what I experienced with the green lady. The worst part of the whole experience for me was the realization that she had eventually to go away. To feel the level of connection and communion that I felt in the presence of the green lady, only to realize that it must end, created a conflict in me that was almost unbearable. It was for me a taste of heaven, and I felt that I could live for a thousand years if I could somehow preserve the strength I felt in the communion with her. The pain of the realization that the connection with the green lady was to be only temporary was for me compounded by the fact that soon after initiation I was told that to fulfill my purpose I must also leave my community to live in the West.

Despite my sorrow, my experience left me with the feeling and the realization that if I am truly connected to my community, that community becomes a form of immortality. For the Dagara people, death results in simply a different form of belonging to the community. It is a lesson from nature that change is the norm, that the world is defined by eternal cycles of decline and regeneration. Having journeyed adequately in this world in your life, you become much more effective to the community that contained you when you return to the world of Spirit. When my grandfather, Bakhyè, died, he told my father, "I have to go now. From where I'll be I'll be more useful to you than if I stay here." Death is not a separation but a different form of communion, a higher form of connectedness with the community, providing an opportunity for even greater service. The kind of connection that I felt with the green lady made me feel as if I could never really die, that I could face any danger or violence and that nothing would ever harm me. The consequence of this feeling was a change in my perception of death. How could it any longer be frightening? Even in death we are connected to the community.

ANCESTORS AND NATURE

When people die, nature is the only hospitable place where their spirits can dwell. Their spirits, living on in the Other World, remember clearly the experience of walking on the earth. They remember the moments when they contributed to greater good and helped to make the world better. But they also remember with great remorse the failed adventures and the gestures that harmed others and made the world a less dignifying place. The more they see this the more they ache, and the more they ache the more eager they are to turn their attention to helping those still in this world. To be active in this world, however, spirits need to enlist our cooperation and help.

In order to crack open something in yourself to allow you to be aware of the presence of ancestors' spirits, you have to walk into nature with your emotional self, not with your intellectual self. You need to open wide your heart so that you can become moist and drink deeply from the emotional echoes that you receive from the frown of a gnarled tree or the twist of a branch. Seen in this way, nature, the dwelling place of the ancestral spirits, is a vast field of grief. I say this because every harmful thing done to the earth is registered in nature. Nature is the place where the real work of healing takes place slowly and gradually. This is because nature cannot ignore the wounds that humans inflict on one another and on her. If nature is the only hospitable place that can hold the spirits that leave the cities and towns, then it is beyond thought what will happen if nature, already so endangered, is destroyed. As part of the healing that we all deserve and all need, the natural world calls us to enter in and allow our grieving self to commune with what already exists there. When there is a grief ritual in my village, it happens in nature, in the open air, not in a church or in some clean, well-lit building. Grieving takes place among the trees, because grief is exactly the sort of thing that the trees will echo and the earth will absorb most naturally. The expression of grief in the presence of nature brings not only healing, but in the end a much stronger connection with nature and the spirits in nature that witness us.

Rituals, such as grieving, are activities that evoke our emotional self. And ritual itself is one of the roads to experiencing the other dimensions of nature through the recognition that one carries within oneself an emotional heritage, an emotional gift. When there is a place for people to listen to the voice of their own emotions, it leads to the opening of a wider door that can allow people to start communing. Communion happens when the emotional body is involved, when we enlist the kind of energy that is expressed in emotional intensity. Imagine the climate of emotional intensity that surrounds a stadium during the Super Bowl; then imagine what it would be like to carry this same intensity of emotion on an individual level into an interaction with a natural place that is untouched by modern technology. You begin to see how you might alter your perception of that natural place. An approach to nature that is accompanied by emotion begins to open the door that will allow communion, for emotion is the key that can open a person to seeing what is present in the natural world. Feeling is the motor of action. It is the fire that moves us into doing things. It is also the teacher of human wisdom.

CULTIVATING A RELATIONSHIP WITH NATURE

It is more important to heal our relationship with nature by doing our own emotional work than by seeking extraordinary experiences that appear supernaturally powerful. Shedding our own tears of grief for the violence done to nature and for the alienation and losses we have experienced in our lives will open the doors to healing faster than will searching for little people who live in another dimension. For however much we are attracted to the Other World revealed in nature, we must understand that if nature were to strip itself naked and appear to us as it is while we are at our present level of consciousness, we would behave in exactly the same way as if God were to come to Earth and walk among us. The stock market would crash, and society would fall apart.

The fear and chaos that would result would be like what happened in a recent event in my West Coast city. It occurred during the Chinese New Year celebration. People in a dragon costume went to visit an elementary school, intending to share a joyous cultural tradition with the students. Instead, the dragon scared the children tremendously, creating a frightening level of panic and confusion. I was very moved, for as I watched the news report of this incident, I saw exactly what it would be like if the spirits from the Other World showed themselves to us continuously through nature, fulfilling our wish to see them. We would find ourselves feeling sorry for having asked for something and gotten it.

The presence of Spirit and the Other World that we encounter in nature can be somewhat scary, and every time people get close to it you can tell that they are not quite comfortable. Indeed, my mother was anxious when I disappeared after following the *kontomblé* that looked like a rabbit into the bush not only because she had lost her son for an entire day, but because she knew of people who had gone to the place I had been who had never come back. The spirits that live in the Other World will tell people who say that they want to see them that if they were to show themselves the way they are, it would disrupt everything in their life, creating more chaos than they could handle. The spirits from the Other World are very careful about not intruding, as though they have laws that forbid them from interfering too much with the normal progress of human beings lest they alter our natural future. Even with all the knowledge I have and all the witnessing I have done of beings from the Other World, coming face-to-face with them, talking with them, triggers such emotion in me that now they have to hide themselves from me. When I am with my sister, who works with helper spirits, and she invites them to come and be present, I stay in the next room, choosing not to visit with them myself, knowing that too much havoc will be created.

My sister's helping spirits are constantly telling her specific things to do that will help restore balance to situations that need healing. She might be asked to perform a specific ritual in a very specific place in a very specific manner. Rituals such as this have a powerful effect on individuals, as if they rebuild us at the level of our cells, allowing us to be more receptive to the reality of the world of Spirit that we are trying to merge with. In the rest of the book we will be exploring rituals in more detail. Here it is important to emphasize that rituals, for indigenous people, grow out of their relationship with nature and the healing, both individual and communal, that takes place through that relationship.

For those of us who are not called to work directly with the spirits, our work consists in healing relationships where we experience separation and brokenness. We can begin this work by reconnecting, in the first place, with the natural world. For nature is our first home, the foundation of the community, the dwelling place of the spirits who watch over us and long to be reconnected with us.

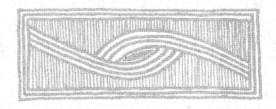

3.

Indigenous Technologies

Where is the Life we have lost in living?
Where is the wisdom we have lost in knowledge?
Where is the knowledge we have lost
in information?
The cycles of Heaven in twenty centuries
Bring us farther from God and nearer to the Dust.
—T. S. ELIOT, "The Rock"

Rooted in nature as the Dagara people are, we have developed forms of technology—of interacting with the natural world—that preserve the delicate balances of the environment and that serve human needs. In the West, technology is usually defined as applying knowledge to serve a practical purpose; among the Dagara and many other tribal cultures, technology is what keeps the individuals and the relationships between individuals and nature healthy. Though Western culture aims at improving the quality of life (and has accomplished this, at least as far as the eye can see), these improvements have come at a price: humans have become indebted to their technology. To indigenous people, the individual in the West has been made a servant to technology; in the indigenous world, by contrast, technologies serve the individual.

Technologies in the indigenous world do not enslave people, because they include the world of Spirit. Perhaps because of that, indigenous technology is accomplished not by machines, but by a dynamic interplay among the mind, emotion, spirit, and senses of the human body on the one hand, and the natural world on the other. In the indigenous world, the physical human constitution is regarded as an expression of mind and Spirit, and a rather limited expression at that. The material world appears quite rigid and constrained compared to the expansive and dynamic energetic world from which it arises. Therefore indigenous technology concerns not only the material world but extends to and grows out of our interaction with Spirit; it is the embodying of our relationship with Spirit.

Since indigenous technologies incorporate the world of Spirit, they often look magical and supernatural to Western eyes. But Western science and technology also have their elements of mystery and magic. In the office of a Silicon Valley engineer, for instance, I saw a poster that declared, "Any technology, sufficiently advanced, appears magical." What may be difficult for the Western mind to accept is the sophistication of a technology that includes so little machinery. But indigenous people are committed to interacting with the natural world without consuming resources; they have developed techniques that work—and appear to work efficiently—precisely because they interact with the realm of Spirit as well.

This is not a polemic intended to foster dislike of modern technologies, replacing them with a worship of indigenous ones. Rather, the purpose here is to open a window of reconciliation between two cultures' ways of responding to the world. What indigenous and Western peoples have in common is the desire to understand the intricacies and complexities of the world we live in and to harness the power of nature for certain practical purposes. Where we have taken different routes, however, is the context within which we have developed our technologies and the purposes for which we have used them. In the West, technology is oriented toward industrial, commercial, and military uses; among indigenous people, it serves to heal and help people remember and fulfill their purpose in life.

In this chapter, then, we will look at how matter and Spirit interact in the indigenous world to form technology. We will look at the place of technology in the work worlds of the Dagara, and we will discuss the purposes for which indigenous technologies are used.

MATTER AND SPIRIT

In the cosmology of the Dagara peoples, matter and Spirit are fused. These two phenomena are complementary, each a reflection of the other. In the Dagara story of creation, the physical world that we can touch and feel and see came into being in parallel with a brighter, more dynamic and expansive energetic world that we call the Other World, or the Spirit World, or the unseen world. These two aspects of the universe do not exist as a polarity, for each is a manifestation of the other, and each is dependent on the other, with a stream of interaction going both ways to maintain balance and stability. The indigenous belief of the Dagara is that we are primarily Spirit. In order to exist as material beings, we have to take a form, and there is the sense among my people that to be in matter is not the most familiar or suitable form for us. To fit ourselves into the narrow part of the universe that allows energy to exist as matter takes some getting used to, and we only bother with it at all because it serves the useful and unavoidable purpose of expanding the spirit in us. It's as if in order to expand or to grow, one must contract or squeeze. The contracted form of our volatile spirit is the body. The adventures of the body prepare the spirit for the leap into its next phase of growth.

The connection to Spirit and the Other World is a dialogue that goes two ways. We call on the spirits because we need their help, but they need something from us as well. We feed something back to them that they need. It is crucial to understand that we are not impotent, we are not creatures that are so helpless that our resources at the level of our spirit have to be entirely delivered from somewhere else.

The world of spirit constantly intrudes on our daily lives, trying to find ways to attract our attention to them, simply because our awareness brings benefits that are good for them. They look at us as an extension of themselves, and so as a result, their own extension must be made either to grow up to the level of vision that they have, or must be adjusted in one way or another so as to keep continuity on their side. There is in this context a mutual interest in having the world we live in and the world of Spirit in harmony. Seen in this way, the benefit that comes to us directly is a recognition of our own sacredness. If we are an object of interest by beings that we consider sacred and spiritual, then that means that we are valuable to them, in the same way that some of us think that they are valuable to us.

There is a reciprocity here that really cancels out the whole sense of hierarchy. If Spirit is looking up to us, and we are looking up to Spirit, then we are looking up to each other, and human beings should take from this a certain sense of dignity. This is an important idea, because the same sense of hierarchy is found in the thinking of some Westerners that romanticizes the indigenous world and indigenous life, or in the thinking of indigenous peoples that romanticize the material abundance of the industrialized world. The industrialized world and the indigenous world need to look up to each other.

I must not discount the importance of things material in Western culture, or even in indigenous culture. People's attraction to material things is proportional to their thirst for the source from which the things come. Think, for example, of a bubbling spring of water. Modern people want to install pipes and bring the water home through a faucet. Indigenous people prefer to leave the spring as it is and to go there when they need it. In this case, indigenous cultures are viewing matter through the lens of

Spirit, whereas in modern culture, Spirit is seen through the lens of matter. It often seems that people in the West go to church on Sundays to excuse themselves from having to worry about Spirit for the next six days while they pursue matter in a very determined way.

What does matter look like when viewed through the lens of Spirit? Matter looks a veil, obscuring the brighter world of Spirit. Or it looks like skin, existing on the boundary between the exterior and the interior of the body. To indigenous people, matter is the skin of Spirit, a permeable boundary between the dimensions.

Imagine that you are a person in Africa who is deeply spiritual and who needs to go out and find a job. You wouldn't begin in the common way that people begin in the West, first obtaining and gathering qualifications and credentials. Instead, you would go first to the shaman, and there you would say, "I'm going to look for a job, and I want the help Spirit to find it." The shaman in his divination will check with the spirits and find out what it is that you are meant to do. Frequently you will be asked to make certain kinds of giveaways and perform certain kinds of rituals, most of them very simple, such as making an offering to Spirit in return for a request for abundance and physical security. Notice here that something must be given first before anything is received. After the giving, then you go into the job market and look for a job like everybody else. What you find is that where the window of opportunity is small, as in the case of tough competition, it becomes much easier to navigate, because you have an invisible spiritual support that others may not have, and this is a credential that very few employers can pass up. Eventually you do get where you want to be, but with a lot less stress, simply because you know that you are not alone in what you are doing; you have had help. If you approached such a task on your own, with only the resources you could bring to the task, then you would have to compete hard in order to succeed. Consequently the shaman, who is in effect a career counselor with information from the Other World of the ancestors, is helpful at more than one level. He does not just tell you what job to look for, he tells you what Spirit wants you to do in order to qualify for the job that befits you.

The resources of the material world may appear scarce and unavailable. So you have to solicit help from a different dimension in order to find and domesticate them. This implies that there needs to be a relationship between matter and Spirit. For when Spirit can manifest things, they last and nourish the soul of the recipient, not merely the body.

Matter is to us as the shadow of a tree is to the tree. Matter looks like the shadow of something real, and for the indigenous mind, the thing from which the shadow originates is more interesting and more worthy of attention than the shadow itself. I cannot look at myself and think that I am seeing the real thing, for a shadow cannot be the source of itself.

Important in this discussion is an understanding of the difference between visibility and invisibility, between the seen and the unseen. We perceive the world based on our expectations, which are heavily determined by our context. If your background or culture has convinced you that what is real is only what is palpable and physical and that seeing is believing, then you will begin to subscribe to what Dagara people call the narrowest horizon of vision. What you see will be based on an internal programming that expects the things of the world to present themselves in ways that you expect so as not to disrupt your entire belief system. Even things that are highly spiritual will have to align themselves with this limited expectation that you have. The narrower your perception, the less accessible to Spirit it is.

The nature ritual I engaged in during my initiation of gazing at a tree and seeing the green lady greatly expanded my own vision. I learned that though my eyes could see perfectly, still my vision could be improved, for there is more to sight than just physical seeing. Nature places only a thin veil over its true self, yet it is a veil that our physical vision cannot penetrate. After my experience with the green lady, I perceived that we are often watched at close distance by spirits that we ourselves do not see, and that when we do see the otherworldly spirits, it is only after they have given us permission to see further—and only after they have made some adjustment in themselves to present themselves to us in ways that preserve their integrity.

This is an extremely important subject, for we cannot assume that people either have to or do see the same things. My people have many words for *vision;* the Dagara want to distinguish between a perception that honors the shadow of Spirit, which here in the West is called ordinary perception or perception of the material world, and the perception of the vital spirit of things, which lies behind the shadow. The shadow has a type of substance such that other shadows can approach it and see it. However, if you are looking only for shadows you will see only shadows; to see Spirit you must revert to your spiritual sight. This is similar to what in the West is called ecstatic perception.

What I saw in my initiation was the result of a struggle that resulted in the aligning of my physical vision with my spiritual sight. This is one way of explaining how a tree changed into a large green woman. In the same way, my meeting the *kontomblé* in the rabbit depended on the fact that my perception as a child had not yet been tampered with or tempered by very earthly things. The spiritual eye that was willing to see the Spirit World had not yet become clouded. I was not surprised when I saw a rabbit turn into a tiny man telling me that the rabbit was my brother. However electrifying the experience was, it was not scary to me, and in fact it seemed quite reasonable and natural at the time. There is some sense in which a child's perception has greater room for spirituality, for spiritual perception.

Indigenous technology is best approached from the context of spiritual perception. For when we see with spiritual eyes, we remain in service to nature; we see nature as the originator of our tools, and we know that our tools or our technology must be used in harmony with nature's design and purposes, which are to maintain and serve the individual and community. Indigenous people approach technology with a mind that is not antagonistic to the whole of things, to communion between the natural and the spiritual. Also, they want to make sure that the individual's work is contributing not only to the individual but also to the collective or the community. It is as if the job that I do is a gift both to me and the people around me. My work responds to nature's expectation of me as a product of nature, rather than something I do in the interest of accumulating or consuming.

What is the relationship between Spirit and the technological? This is an invitation to consider that there is something technological in spirituality, as there is something spiritual in technology. A harmonious relationship between Spirit and technology begins with trust in one's vision and one's perception. It proceeds through believing that what is commonly regarded as fantasy is not impossible, for instance that someone who dreams of becoming a bird can actually become one provided that he or she works at it and believes it as a reality. Our vision is the starting point of a primal technological power, which is the ability to manifest, to make Spirit real in material form.

BODY AND SPIRIT AT WORK

Spirit and work are linked among indigenous people because human work is viewed as an intensification of the work that Spirit does in nature. Spirit administers nature, the complex interweaving of life forms and cycles of time that we experience as the natural world. Nature, in fact, is such a complex organism that only the intelligence of Spirit can manage it.

Individuals, as extensions of Spirit, come into the world with a purpose. At its core, the purpose of an individual is to bring beauty, harmony, and communion to Earth. Individuals live out their purpose through their work. Thus the human work of maintaining the world, to indigenous people, is an extension of the work that Spirit does to maintain the pulse of nature. The villager's quest for wholeness is an extension of nature's wholeness.

How do villagers arrive at wholeness, at the happy goal of realizing their purpose and contributing to the healing of this world? By emphasizing service, community, and dedication to individual vision. Dedicating themselves to these values, indigenous people maintain an intimate connection between their work and the products of their work—a connection that for the industrialized West has been severed, as Marx was the first to note. For villagers, the product of any work must be engineered not only to serve the collective good but also to be an extension of the goodness of the collective.

For instance, when women get together to make pottery, they are acknowledging that their ability to create is a part of nature's design, a part of their purpose. Before a woman participates in the work with clay, which is the earth, she will first gather the signs and images she has seen in nature, and she will bring these signs into the circle of other women. In the interest of producing something that is an extension of their wholeness, the women will begin by chanting and singing together, echoing one another. The work is not in the form of a production line, even though a production line would have yielded more than enough of these practical containers. Nor do the women work alone. Each person has clay. They are seated in a circle, and they chant until they are in some sort of ecstatic place, and it is from that place that they begin molding the clay. It is as if the knowledge of how to make pots is not in their brains, but in their collective energy. The product becomes an extension of the collective energy of the circle of women.

I have watched this process unfold countless times. The women can sit all day in front of two dozen mounds of clay, doing nothing but chanting—until the last hours, when in a flurry of activity all kinds of pots come forth. Imagine a job where two-thirds of the time was spent chanting, and one third was spent in production! The product of work here, the pot, embodies the intimacy and wholeness experienced by the women over the course of the day. The women understand that it is necessary to reach that place of wholeness before they can bring something out of it.

Farming works in the same way. We don't just farm. We have to be able to invoke the kind of power that can come only from the natural world and to bring it to bear on the work we are doing. Only then can the nourishment that is pulled from the land have lasting consequences and lasting effects.

As a result of our work practices, the indigenous notion of abundance

is very different from that in the West. Villagers are interested not in accumulation but in a sense of fullness. Abundance means a sense of fullness, which cannot be measured by the yardstick of the material goods we
possess or the amount of money in a bank account. Abundance, in that
sense of fullness, has a power that takes us away from worry. It is the kind
of feeling you get when you are in communion with the natural, in communion with the source. There is some sense in which the work, or the
love of work, is the love of this kind of abundance. It is the kind of fullness you get by being with other people. Most work done in the village is
done collectively. The purpose is not so much the desire to get the job
done but to raise enough energy for people to feel nourished by what they
do. The nourishment does not come *after* the job, it comes *before* the job
and *during* the job. The notion that you should do something so that you
get paid so that then you can nourish yourself disappears. You are nourished first, and then the work flows out of your fullness.

Many areas of work among villagers, including farming, are accompanied by music. Music is meant to maintain a certain state of fullness.
People recognize that even if you are full before the work, you can't take
that fullness for granted. You have to keep feeding it so that the feeling of
fullness continues, so that the work you are doing constantly reflects that
fullness in you. It is as if the output of work takes a toll on your fullness,
even if it is an expression of your fullness, and you have to be filled again
before you can continue. Music and rhythm are the things that feed someone who is producing something.

Work in my village thus is structured very differently from the way it
is structured in the West, and yet the completed product has the same
pride attached to it. Work, in an indigenous context, becomes dominated
by art. It is as if art is the ideal tool fusing body, Spirit, and work. To grow
and harvest a yam takes more than know-how. It must include style,
beauty, and the embracing of the spirit of yam.

There is an intimate relationship in an indigenous village between art
and ritual. What the workers are doing is essentially a ritual, and that ritual heals them. It produces a healed self by showing them evidence of

what they are; they are mirrored in the product that has flowed out of them. I remember my mother uttering very moving, poetic chants as she milled grain, grinding for six hours to fill only a small bucket. The meal that came out of her work contained tremendous energy, the spiritual energy of the poetry and music as well as the physical energy contained in the grain. All of her work was a work of art, done so genuinely, with total devotion, that it contributed to a profound sense of fullness in the family.

Peoples' relationships are cemented in the work, because in some way the product and the collective chanting weave a thread among the people, bringing them even closer to one another. The work is a ritual. The product, and the technology, is art.

Readers may be wondering how this harmonious picture of villagers chanting and singing together as they shape pots or grow yams fits with the more common pictures they have been shown of African children starving and of the grim specter of death bearing down upon tribal communities. What I must emphasize here is that the energy required to sustain the harmony we are talking about is so delicate that it can easily be destroyed by the slightest intrusion, and such intrusion has clearly taken place through colonialism. Africa today is not what it used to be. The point for me is not to speak about the lack of dignity evidenced by the images of starvation. These images have cemented a certain stereotype of Africans, a stereotype created by the destruction wrought through colonialism.

When colonialism, old or new, disrupts the energy working like an umbrella to protect people, the people under the umbrella will be exposed to the elements. Like fish in a lake whose water has suddenly evaporated, the fish will die. The great problem is that the fish have been brought to public attention after the drying of the lake; beholders may not remember the fish as it was or could have been in a full lake. Thus Western perception of African tribal life has been heavily influenced by a media more interested in negative sensationalism than in images of beauty and harmony. What I want to communicate in this book is what I assume most

Westerners don't know about indigenous ecology. I may not be able to counteract the images of Africa already seared into the memory of the average Westerner. But I might at least bang at the door of a cultural fundamentalism that has prevented the images of the village as I know it from reaching the eyes of Westerners.

TECHNOLOGY AND THE NATURAL WORLD

In the indigenous world, technology takes a radically different form than in the West because its intention is not to disturb the natural world. Indigenous people tend to be familiar with the sorts of technology that do not assault nature, do not compete with the natural order, and do not tend to show them as superior with respect to nature. This does not imply that villagers are not interested in learning to manipulate Western technology, but for the most part their interest is matched by ignorance of how it works and how to relate to it. The chief of a village is awarded a moped, the equivalent of a limousine in the modern world. He is delighted by this gesture of respect. A few days later he is found in the middle of the bush pushing the bike and cursing. Asked what happened, he says the damn thing just stopped and decided to stay there. He decides that this gift was nothing more than a trick to humiliate him in front of his people. The chief was only out of gas and did not know it. So if the poor man can't tell when his moped is out of gas, how many more griefs await him when he bypasses the recommended maintenance schedule?

Indigenous technology, which focuses on working with the world of Spirit, requires the same awareness for safe operation as does Western technology focused on manipulating matter. To African villagers, the skills of working with the world of Spirit arise as a gift from nature, given for the good of people. Technology is seen in this context as the vehicle for going home, because once you have your hand on these technologies you are reminded that your true home is out there somewhere, somewhere else, and it makes you want to get there fast. It doesn't make you want to settle in here with a mountain of possessions and a large mortgage. The true indigenous technology is aimed at returning people to their origin, returning people to where they came from, the Spirit World.

Technologies in the indigenous world are developed in order to fulfill basic human needs, such as community, health, harmony, and a sense of meaning and purpose in life. In this sense technology is oriented toward Spirit. This seems to contrast with the West, where the craving for connection with a deeper sense of meaning and the yearning for spiritual vitality are mostly diluted amid the noise of traffic and factories. Yet it is obvious that the one wants or needs the other. Villagers in West Africa who are taken on a tour of a factory often come out of there silent for days, unable to put in words what they saw. They are mesmerized at the power of the machine and its ability to make things. Some are confused as to whether there is a spirit behind all this or if the machine is not the spirit in disguise. They report that they feel as if their spirit was sucked out in the factory and that they need healing to recover from their encounter. This recovery often leads to the person returning to the city in search of the god of the white man whose power they have seen. But enchantment with technology can work in the other direction also. A Westerner is introduced to village "magic" and decides to settle there. Every year I am aware that many people take off to my village because they read about the magic of Dagara people.

The challenge in sharing or explaining indigenous technologies to Westerners is similar to the challenge of explaining modern technologies to indigenous people. Could this be part of the reason why Third World countries have a hard time developing in the modern way? Modern farming systems that have been imported to Africa, including sophisticated machinery and fertilizers, have created more problems than they have resolved. Over a decade ago, French people introduced cotton farming to my village as a cash-producing industry so that villagers might buy Western products such as bicycles, shortwave radios, and clothing. Those who participated in the program will never forget the disaster they brought to themselves and their families. In order to grow cotton, they had to do so as the French taught—by purchasing fertilizer and DDT on credit. By the time the crop was harvested, the land had "died," or as villagers say, the earth spirit had become angry. The sale of the cotton barely reimbursed the cost of the fertilizer and pesticide, and the families of those who had hoped to profit had to turn for support to the families who did not participate in the program. People cried out that modern technology had come in to devour their spirit. Things have improved since then, allowing people to participate in a more educated way in the agricultural revolution. But whom has this revolution benefited? Which of the world's growing populations have been fed? Indigenous people see that food has flowed to the modern world more than to the indigenous world.

Many ecologists and environmentalists in the West say that technology sets itself up as an enemy of nature. They fight to close a nuclear power plant here or there because they understand that the purity of Nature is being contaminated by these plants, and the consequences to countless species, including humankind, are serious. Westerners talk about rivers of pure water having become like sewers. One gets an image of industry abandoning its droppings anywhere it wishes, knowing full well that what it cannot digest, nothing can. Some suggest this is the price to pay to get the results needed. Hasn't modern technology, overall, contributed to bettering human life? The problem is that wherever there is a yet-undamaged piece of the world, modernity tends to regard that place as primitive, archaic, and, at best, preindustrial.

By contrast, indigenous technologies look rather nonaggressive. In producing anything, indigenous people make it a point to inquire with the Spirit World as to whether this product is appropriate. Usually it is, otherwise the idea would never have come to their consciousness to begin with. For indigenous Africans, dream and vision are evidence of the Spirit pointing the way to us. What is shown to you in that manner is actually an invitation from a higher realm to consecrate yourself to the production of something that is going to benefit the greater community.

TECHNOLOGIES OF THE PHYSICAL WORLD:
HERBAL MEDICINE

Certain indigenous technologies look superficially like Western scientific technology. The use of certain herbal medicines resembles Western pharmacology, with some herbs having objective indications that are the same for most people, such as certain plants that women take for birth control, or specific plant medicines that are used widely to treat dysentery, tuberculosis, and other infectious diseases and parasites. But what is it about the way that pharmacology is approached in the village that is connected to Spirit? It would appear that any herbalist could conjure a formula, knowing that if you have this symptom, you can take such and such herb. Yet traditional indigenous herbal medicine functions in a way that is different, not only from Western allopathic or herbal medicine, but also from Oriental herbal medicine. For indigenous herbal medicine incorporates the seeking of Spirit in the administering of all substances.

According to indigenous African philosophy, you cannot just give an aspirin or cook up an herbal recipe for the purpose of healing. There are two things at work. One is the knowledge of the spiritual nature of the plants, and the second and more important is the knowledge of the energetic configuration and the identity and purpose of the person you are treating. It is not the illness possessing the person that is important, but the person possessing the illness. In an indigenous view of illness, the disease is always linked to a breakage in relationship. Some connection is loose or completely absent, or has been severed. What the villager sees in the physical disease is simply the aftermath of something that has happened on the level of energy or relationship. The illness is a physical manifestation of a spiritual decay.

Treating the illness, in the indigenous view, means conjuring up an energy that will repair the spiritual state so that the spiritual healing can be translated into healing of the physical disease. You have to heal in the Spirit World before you can heal in the physical world. The physical illness is simply a shadow of the spiritual dysfunction that exists. In any attempt to heal, it is good to know a few herbs, but it is better to know the energetic background of the patient and the reason for the physical illness.

Once the energetic background of the illness is known, then one has to move to the next stage, which has to do with getting the plants, the roots, and the leaves to cooperate in bringing the repaired energy from the spiritual world across to the physical world to heal the body. For cooperating in this way is precisely what plants do; they are one vehicle through which a repaired state of affairs is extended into the physical world. How do indigenous people haul this healing across into the physical world? First, the healer has to know the time and place of the birth of the person, to narrow the range of plants that will contribute to that person's healing. Then the healer usually goes out on the person's birthday to collect the plants needed. (In Dagara medicine, a person's birthday occurs once every five days, since everyone is said to have an affinity with one of the five days of the Dagara weekly cycle.) Certain people possess natural healing powers that include the use of plants gathered in a specific order. What they know is easily knowable by anybody, yet it seems that they alone can produce the desired result. This is why it appears that Spirit has something to do with healing.

The spiritual, the supernatural in a sense, seems to be the supervising force of indigenous pharmacology, to the point that it looks as though without the Spirit nothing works. This is why, in an extreme case, you might see a healer just grab some dirt and feed it to someone in acute distress, and the crisis that person was in will stop immediately. You know when you see it that you cannot replicate that yourself. I was once a witness when an old woman went suddenly into a seizure that ended in a coma. A healer was present who immediately took a dipper of water in a gourd and added some of the dirt from the woman's last footprint. He was wearing a ring, which he added to the mix, and the mix started to froth and boil. He removed the ring and left instructions that all of the contents of the gourd had to make it into her belly. As soon as the woman's family managed to get the mud into her, she woke up, looking surprised and asking what happened. Such events signify to indigenous people that Spirit is supervising the healing procedure, for to indigenous people as well as Westerners, these are not everyday occurrences that can be replicated by just anyone. Spirit works through the healer to create the exact medicine that will bring the healing appropriate to this particular patient and situation.

TECHNOLOGIES OF THE SPIRITUAL WORLD: GATEWAYS

For healing to last, the healed energy in the spiritual plane must be brought across to the physical world. This is done by bringing it through a gateway between the spiritual and material worlds. What is the gateway? A gateway is a door to the Spirit realm that is connected to a particular place in the physical world. Healers who bring energy from the Spirit World through the gateways are known as gatekeepers. A gatekeeper can trace the shadow from this world back to its origin in the spiritual world and act as an intermediary, as a bridge, since he or she understands the relationship between the different aspects of the reality of this world.

The gateways that are maintained in certain places in nature are themselves important technologies for healing. Technologies such as this are viewed as magical and supernatural and are therefore suspect, sometimes frightening, to the Western mind. But recall the Silicon Valley poster, "Any technology, sufficiently advanced, appears magical." Gateways to the Spirit World may appear magical to Westerners because there is so little hardware involved. Indigenous people value efficiency, and anything that can be accomplished by manipulating energy without consuming resources is preferred.

Their reaction to an episode of *Star Trek* illustrates this perspective. On one of my trips to my village I brought a VCR, a small TV, and some videotapes of this popular science fiction show. During one of the scenes where people were being dematerialized and moved around by the transporter machine, I asked the elders if they understood what was going on. They were rather taken aback, replying that of course they knew what was happening, but could I please explain what all of the machines were for.

A gateway to the Spirit World located in a cave was the technology that provided healing for one of my nieces. My twelve-year-old niece had some strange illness that translated mostly in the form of visions and nightmares. People thought she hallucinated. I was in the village at the time and heard about a new healer in town. I myself needed to visit the healer for a problem that was brewing in my own life. Having a moped at my disposal at the time, I decided to take my little niece on a ride to the healer's. When we arrived, there was quite a crowd. It was late afternoon. He was in his consultation room. I was told that we first needed to see him so that he could determine whether we needed to go to the cave or not. I hoped strongly to be admitted to the cave. So I was very relieved when he announced that both my niece and I needed to join the others for the journey to the cave.

When we arrived there, it was dark. The healer, who was the gatekeeper, came and disappeared into the dark mouth of the grotto without any flashlight. He remained there for quite some time before coming out. Standing in front of the cave, he made a long prayer, which was punctuated by noises coming out of the cave. It was as if people were talking back at him, and things were moving very fast just inside the opening. Eventually a faint light came out of the cave and settled there. He turned around, and said, "They are here, just get in one at a time." Almost half of the people declined the offer. My niece's jaws were clacking with fear, and her knees were knocking against each other. I encouraged her to enter the cave because nothing bad was going to happen to her. Meanwhile people entered the cave and came out with little packages in their hands. My turn came, and I went in. I was met by a tiny female *kontomblé* with rolling eyes. She asked me to wait because she was going to get something at home for me. Then she disappeared into thin air. I was used to the *kon-*

tomblé, so I was not impressed. Ten seconds or less later, she showed up smiling and carrying something in her baby hands. She spoke a language I did not understand, but she was beckoning me to come closer. When she put the medicine into my hands, I happened to touch her tiny fingers. They were cold, not of this world.

When I walked out, it was my niece's turn. I encouraged her one last time. Hesitantly she walked in. It felt like an eternity waiting for her because I could feel every bit of her fear. I heard a screeching sound, and my heart stopped, then I felt very calm and content. I knew my niece was okay. When she came out, she had nothing in her hands. Her face was beaming with joy. She said she had met her friends, the very people she saw in her hallucinations. They were happy that she had come home to them finally, and they said they were going to work with her. She said one of them, a woman, took her on a ride on her back. They went far into a beautiful landscape. They were flying up and down hills and mountains while she kept telling her not to be afraid because this is her home. And so she felt no fear. She did not remember how to be afraid, it was so beautiful. She was crying. I felt her joy while we rode home. The villagers understand that this special connection with the *kontomblé* and the Spirit World held by my niece is a gift, and she will have a mentor who will help her hold and develop this gift in a way that will be healing for her and the others in the village.

Readers may be wondering if insights from indigenous medicine might be efficacious in the Western world. I wonder if cases of mental illness, of the phenomenon known as chemical imbalance, and even depression might not be cases that could be addressed in this manner. For even the possibility that some mental or emotional imbalance could be the prelude to a better and brighter life, as were my niece's "hallucinations," might act like medicine, restoring hope in a situation that appears unresolvable. While gatekeepers and *kontomblé* may not be available to Westerners, perhaps some form of collective ritual could draw Spirit into such cases. We will speak of specific healing and communal rituals later in the book.

CHANGE AND EVOLUTION

A culture that is in touch with its spiritual connection is a culture that is poised to evolve. In the indigenous context, change is tolerated, even welcomed, because it originates with Spirit. If evolution originates in a spiritual source, then it does not disrupt stability. If evolution is seen in terms of the modern definition, concerned with ascendancy, acquisition, and control and mastery over the material world, then evolution becomes destructive to stability. The modern notion of stability has a heavy load of military hardware associated with it. This contrasts sharply with the indigenous view of stability, which is a state of alignment with Spirit, with cosmic rules and regulations.

The very word *cosmos* implies evolution, and in this context, evolution means discovering new things and learning new methods of handling the affairs of life. This is one purpose of technology, to help human beings increase their awareness and consciousness. In this sense precolonial indigenous cultures, even within their apparently primitive technologies, were heavily involved in an evolutionary process. In the interest of their own evolution, it was essential to maintain cohesion within the culture, for you have to stick together to evolve together. In the development of Western technologies, we cannot allow some among us to evolve while some are left behind, because that is not community. Community is the common handling of the journey. Attention to community and to Spirit in indigenous technologies has meant, however, that the evolution of indigenous cultures takes place quietly, without the explosive and destructive side effects of Western technology. When your ties with Spirit are strong enough, your evolution has less visibility. A good portion of modern technology is extremely destructive, probably because of the lesser presence of Spirit within it. The larger the presence of the Spirit, the subtler and less polluting technological evolution will be.

All of the indigenous technologies we have discussed have the ability to change and adapt, and they usually adjust themselves to changing needs in the community. Before the coming of modernity, the people who were the healers would have others in the village come and work on their farm, and they would always end up with enough food to feed their families. Now that this system no longer exists, you will find a shaman with a tiny yard, and from this he can pull enough food to feed a family of twenty children. This is an evolution in technology, based on drawing the vitality of nature to that tiny plot in order to produce enough food, relying much more on invisible forces such as the blessings you get from nature when you farm.

The reason the shaman's farming has changed is that with the coming of the Western world, even people in the village are losing their interest in the village, and the community there is challenged. People are eager to benefit from the shaman's services, but they no longer want to work on his farm. This prompted a new paradigm, whereby the shaman uses his knowledge to produce the food he needs from a very small plot of land, but there is a consequence for this change, for less of the shaman's energy is available for healing in the village.

The changes that occur in the indigenous technologies do not occur because some shaman sets out to find a better way to do things. Seen with a modern eye, this looks like one of the shortcomings of indigenous culture. For since no one appears to be actively trying to do anything differently, or better, there is the appearance that the culture is stagnant. It is the indigenous understanding, however, that ideas you receive do not come from your imagination, they come from the Spirit World, and it is the spirits who will decide what the next step will be, what changes if any need to be made in the technologies that they have given to you. A person's purpose is to serve, using that which has been put into his or her hands as a gift from Spirit.

Also, the Dagara recognize a close relationship between knowledge and secrecy. Beside the fact that what one knows remains alive through its hiddenness, there is an attitude toward knowledge that to know is to become a guardian of something. To circulate the knowledge given to you by Spirit indiscriminately is harmful. Every time I travel home to Africa I am faced with this issue. My quest for magical knowledge will be met by a laconic response stressing my inability to safeguard the knowledge I am seeking.

The first time I asked villagers what they use to open a doorway to another world, I provoked a sudden wall of silence around me. It was at my home, and I was surrounded by a few elders and diviners who were my distinguished guests. I had invited them partly just to host them, but mostly to discuss questions such as this. The bold idea of writing a book about magical practices, including graphic details about those practices, had occurred to me, and I was eager for their input. After serving them a little meal and a lot of drink and watching them engage in some heated debate about ways of preventing natural fatalities such as accident, loss of luck, and misfortune, I thought the time had come to moderate the debate. So I decided to guide it into the area of magic.

I wanted to address the indigenous access to the Other World because it appears so central to the rhythm of life in the village. So I ventured to ask, "Why is the Other World so important to us?" This question met with many answers. Everyone commented on it, stressing the impossibility of envisioning life without the Other World. This gave me the courage to push further. "How do you open a doorway to the Other World?" I asked, directing the question particularly to one of the diviners who was known in the village as a guardian of the doorways.

The whole room fell silent. My guests looked at one another as if they did not quite understand what I meant. At last the diviner to whom the question was directed replied that I was still a little child in the face of these things. He added, "I myself sometimes feel like a child in front of these things. You see, you are better off not knowing this now, because it will change your life so deeply that you will no longer be able to invite us to drink the white man's drink. This will be disappointing. It is because I know the answer to your question that I spend most of my life out there in the holes of the earth. I don't like it, but I can't forget what I have learned. Cut me some more drink." Saying this, he changed the subject. Out of respect I decided to leave it at that.

Among the Dagara, healing knowledge is usually taught by a being from the Other World, namely a *kontomblé*, or a spirit ally. The viability of the material is verified in the context of the amount of good it does to the village. The healer, that is the technologist, is instrumental to the Spirit's power to heal, and to make changes in human lives. Thus, one can say to a healer, "Teach me what you know"; but the better request to make of the healer is, "Teach me about what teaches you." Since the source, and home, of indigenous technology is nature and the world of Spirit, to that source you must go in order to learn and grow and evolve.

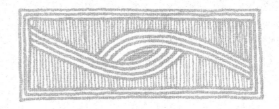

PART TWO

RELATIONSHIPS

OF HEALING:

THE

COMMUNITY

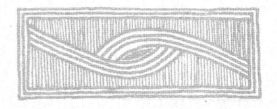

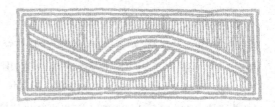

4.

The Value of a
Healthy Community

I celebrate myself, and sing myself,
And what I assume, you shall assume,
For every atom belonging to me
as good as belongs to you.
—WALT WHITMAN, "Song of Myself"

As you land on the single runway of Ouagadougou International Airport after a
five-and-a-half-hour flight that originated
in Paris, you already feel the shock of difference between the hypercomplexity of
modern transport and the blatant barren-
ness of a place that is considered by locals
as the most modern area of the country.
This is because you see it through the eyes
of what you left behind.

As you leave the airport and enter the
city, you may still feel that you are in the

countryside. And when you hit the countryside a few minutes later, you may feel that you are in a truly strange place. Indeed, the sparse trees littering the dry and dusty plain—as if trying to affirm life over desolation—bow at you under the pressure of the *harmattan*, a southwesterly wind triggered by the Sahara Desert sandstorms.

As you drive west on the one-lane road considered to be the nation's main artery, you are plunged into the silence and mystery of the indigenous world. Here, standing on the side of the road, a group of half-naked people, each carrying a large bundle on her or his head, watches you pass in your slow-moving vehicle. You see, they are wondering why you have decided to come to this part of the world. Farther down the road, you have to stop to avoid plowing into a herd of cows and sheep being led slowly across the highway. Minutes later, you may have to get completely off the road to let a cargo truck speed past you, for these trucks own the road. Their only competitors are donkeys hauling a cargo of merchandise, perhaps dry wood, and heading toward the city.

Meanwhile, if you pay attention, you will notice signs that tell you when you are entering a village, but seldom will you notice the village itself. You will see only a hut here and there dispersed amid the trees. This is because you are driving on the main highway. Entrances to these villages are on tiny passageways that lead to the village circle.

After two hundred and twenty kilometers on the tiny paved road, a big sign will appear that tells you to turn left at the next intersection if you intend to enter Dagara land. There ends the leisure of your trip, for the paved road turns to dirt. As you begin riding on it you will think nostalgically about the smooth road you just left. Countless holes that must be avoided at all cost punctuated by spreads of red dirt that turn into a thick cloud of dust as you drive over them make you wonder if you will ever arrive safely at your destination. If you arrive in Dano and ask for the Somé family, people will tell you that half of the area is full of Somés and therefore you will have to be specific. If you are black, you will have to specify which Somé you want, but if you're white, they will know which Somé you are referring to. Either way, you will be the center of a lot of attention because you are a stranger and therefore under the protection of Spirit. If the first person you encounter is a true follower of the tradition, he will take you into his house and ask you to sit and relax. Don't act as if you're in a hurry; he has to fulfill his obligation to Spirit. He will not answer your question as to where the Somés are until refreshment is brought to you. Then he will ask you about your journey. Just say it was good; then he will praise the Spirit for you. After this he will offer to accompany you to where you are going. Do not decline the offer, for it is only traditional for-mality.

When you arrive at your destination with your guide, both of you will be considered as strangers. This is because the one who guides a traveler is also a traveler; Spirit protects both of them. No one will greet you until the water ceremony has been performed first. The water of peace or re-freshment will be brought to the two of you. A drop of it will be poured onto the ground to acknowledge the ancestors. Then the host will sip a lit-tle bit of it before passing it on. You can't say you're not thirsty; this would upset the flow of things. What matters is the symbolism of the ges-ture.

After a long moment of silence, in the course of which you may feel as if you are being ignored, your host will finally come and greet you in person—but only after your guide has told the entire story that explains why you're with him. As your host greets you, people begin to pour in from surrounding compounds, for the news has spread that a stranger has arrived. The greetings may feel interminable to you. After everybody has had a chance to say hello to you, you will be asked to follow the host, along with a few other people, to the ancestral altar. It is often nested in one of the many rooms in a compound or in the front yard. There everybody bends their knees while the host presents the stranger to the ancestors. The host takes some ash on his hand and sprays it on the altar, then speaks of peace, protection, health on behalf of the stranger. After that your guide will leave, promising to return the next day. You will be offered sleeping arrangement after dinner. The reason for your visit will be inquired about only after you have rested. As long as you stay in the village you are cared for as a Spirit envoy and respected. This is the law.

THE VILLAGE COMMUNITY

These elaborate greeting rituals, ending with paying homage at the ancestral altar, reveal something of the customs and values governing the village as a community. The village is organized as a commonwealth under the guidance and supervision of the ancestors, whose laws must be carefully followed to avoid trouble. One of the overarching structures of the village is the clan. In the village every person belongs to a clan that is named after one of the elements of the cosmology. Thus we have water people, fire people, earth people, mineral people, and nature people. (These will be explored more deeply in the chapters that follow.) Each group has a keeper or a chief, and the chief of all the chiefs is the head of the earth group. The chief remains a chief until he dies. Then he is succeeded by someone else in his family. The criteria for the succession is not clear; shamans take care of it in divination. The entire structure is divided along gender lines, allowing male groups to be separate from female groups. Thus the ultimate power base is the council of elders, female and male. Usually there are five of them, corresponding to the five groups.

The responsibility of each chief is to maintain the shrine of the group as well as to ensure that crises are handled the proper way. Each time a crisis occurs between two people, it is resolved by ritual in the presence of everyone else and only after it has been examined through divination to ensure that it is just a conflict and not something deeper affecting more people, like a plague. The parties involved in the conflict come together in an ash circle. They sit facing each other, and the defendant listens to the story of his accuser first. The accuser speaks about how the action of the other made him feel, and the crowd, led by the chief, guides the two parties along. The whole crisis usually ends up looking like an unpleasant misunderstanding, and the two opponents become friends with the applause of everyone witnessing.

Of course things may not always work out like this. It may be that the crisis, because it has been simmering for a long time, does not cool off in the circle of ash. At this point healers are brought in to make an offering to the ancestors so that they can tune up the energies of the two parties in order to allow for a healing ash circle. So a failed ash-circle ritual means that healers have a job to do—to reduce the heat between the two people before they meet again. Should none of this work, it shows that one of the parties is not doing his part. At such a time, the chiefs of all the elements will deliver their warning to the renegade party, making him responsible for the lingering of the crisis.

These crisis resolutions are gender specific. In other words, there is a women's court and a men's court. But there is also ample room for a cross-gender court. Most of the time this court will be used by couples facing the delicate responsibility of keeping their relationship pure by working out the conflicts that arise between them.

In Africa people's welfare and rights are safeguarded by the ancestors. It is the ancestors who ultimately punish wrongdoing, by sending trouble or illness, even death, to the transgressor. When trouble comes, the diviners inquire as to the reason and are able to determine which of the ancestral laws has been broken. In this way abuses are corrected and people are given an opportunity to make amends and turn their lives around.

I recall a time when this process caught up with me. I was involved in a car accident, which turned out to have been sent by the ancestors to prevent me from interfering in a process of growth for my uncle. My uncle was very sick and was being treated at the home of a healer. His disease had debilitated him to the point that he had lost the use of many of his physical abilities. We had been close for years, and upon hearing that I had returned home, my uncle sent a messenger with the request that I give him a ride back to his own home for a few days. I was happy to be of service to a person experiencing great suffering.

The next morning, after very little sleep, I dashed off in a car on the dusty path between villages. After a few minutes I lost control of the car, and the next thing I knew, the car and I had rolled over. I was shaken by the accident and wondered what it might mean. Shamans, upon hearing the news of the accident, performed divinations to find the cause, and their inquiries revealed some disturbing news. According to the ancestors, I should have checked with them to learn why my uncle was sick before running to his aid. His sickness, they said, was a punishment for the violation of family laws, and therefore I could be of no help him.

Apparently more than twenty years earlier, my uncle had treated others in the village quite savagely, creating a lot of upset by being brutal and refusing to sit in ash circles to heal the conflicts he had created. He had been warned of his actions many times, but they had taken place so long ago that most people, including him, had forgotten about the abuses. Yet now, late in his life, when he had softened and changed his ways, his sentence was being meted out to him. In the eyes of the ancestors, a log does not become a crocodile by staying immersed long enough underwater.

I was quite upset by the incident, because the accident could have killed me. Angrily I wondered why no one had told me what was appropriate in the situation. I'd had no idea that a simple human gesture of help, especially toward a family member, should have required a divination. What the experience taught me is that the Dagara culture is changing and that what was once obvious, such as when gestures of support are appropriate, is no longer as clear. These changes gradually seem to separate and isolate the individual from the rest of the community. What I also took from the incident was respect for the way that the community must have cohered in earlier years. Even now, the method of appealing to ancestors for guidance had unearthed abuses buried so long in people's memories that they were no longer visible.

The indigenous method of bringing to light the roots of conflict and illness through communicating with the Spirit World created a coherent and effective circle of support for individuals. Rights were safeguarded and conflicts were resolved with the help of the ancestor spirits. Healing of illness and conflict could take place precisely because the community was defined as including not only human beings but also the spirits of the ancestors, whose vision is broader than that of humans.

THE MODERN SEARCH FOR COMMUNITY

Since coming to the West, I have found that modern people long for the fulfilling connections that are available through a healthy community, the sense of connection and coherence that I have experienced in village life. The cry for community is everywhere. As Carolyn Shaffer and Kristin Anundsen point out in their ambitious and detailed book, *Creating Community Anywhere*, Americans have defined themselves in terms of individual freedom: a people breaking away from old, limiting structures, dogmas, and attitudes and pushing forward to new frontiers. But with every gain there is a loss. *Community* is a term that is so familiar to people in the West and yet so hard to achieve. Constantly on the move from city to city, often separated from one's family by geographical distance, and commonly losing primary relationships, such as marriage, to the ravages of separation, Westerners often find themselves relying solely upon themselves, their distraction of choice, or their therapists to manage the crises of daily living. Meanwhile, their psyches crave belonging in a community with others, where they know they will find healing once and for all.

The urge for community in the West is challenged by the tendency to see community as antithetical, and even a threat, to individuality. Many modern people believe that community absorbs the dignity and integrity of the individual and threatens to kill the much-cherished sense of self. The truth is that one doesn't lose one's self as a result of being part of a community. On the contrary, being in community leads to a healthy sense of belonging, greater generosity, better distribution of resources, and a greater awareness of the needs of the self and the other. In community, the needs of the one are the needs of the many. In community, one does not worry excessively about one's intimate relationships because you are not left to confront your problems alone. In such a context, people are not encouraged to be on the run every day, chasing survival. In this way, being part of a strong community strengthens one's individuality by supporting the expression and enjoyment of one's unique gifts and talents.

Individuality, not individualism, is the cornerstone of community. Individuality is synonymous with uniqueness. This means that a person and his or her unique gifts are irreplaceable. The community loves to see all of its members flourish and function at optimum potential. In fact, a community can flourish and survive only when each member flourishes, living in the full potential of her or his purpose. To honor and support its members is in the self-interest of any community.

WELCOMING CHILDREN INTO COMMUNITY

In my village, people give special attention to the unique potential of each individual—the purpose that each person came into the world to nurture and to make blossom. In order for the community to function in a way that encourages the blossoming of its individuals, indigenous people make every birth a village event, where the newborn is welcomed by all.

I still have vivid images of the most recent birthing ritual I attended in my village. The young mother was in labor all afternoon and was walked around by a group of old women who chanted softly into her ear. The labor must have been very hard on the woman, since she did appear to be in great pain and uninterested in the singing. Yet the songs being sung to her were quite beautiful. They sounded like a litany involving genealogy; ancestors' names were uttered, one after another. Then the women chanted further, and I realized that everything was being said directly to the newborn. Among the most captivating statements were, "You have come to a crossroads. The light you see in front of you is the light of the village that awaits you." Another woman said, "Run, run, run to the gate and do not waste time, because Mummy is in pain." Yet another woman said, "Our great mothers said the walk home used to feel exhausting. But when they found out what was waiting for them at home, they forgot the pain of homecoming. We have sweet grass and honey awaiting your arrival. Sweet bosom ripe with food and love in a hurry to be with you."

At that moment, the laboring woman stopped her pacing. Everyone stopped along with her. The song shifted in theme. It went back to genealogy and stories of valor, then quickly turned into a song of identity. An elder was asking if the unborn remembered what was said a long time ago when he first came into his mother's womb. The verses were meant to be a reminder of the reason why he should be eager for birth.

For the entire afternoon and on until dark, five women gathered and walked with the mother, singing to her unborn all that time. At the time of delivery, the song stopped and the women busied themselves in other work. Meanwhile, children gathered close by, waiting for the big moment. That big moment came when the newborn screamed. Simultaneously, a loud noise bursting out of a dozen children like a tidal wave drowned the screechy sound coming out of the tiny mouth of the newborn. Then everything became quiet. One of the old woman said, "That's a grandfather. Look how he stares at everything." Mother and son were united on the spot and escorted into a dark room, where they would remain hidden for the next seventy-two hours.

I thought to myself that the scream of the newborn had something of a question in it. It was like a signal sent out by the newcomer to see if he had arrived at the right place. The sound most similar to a newborn's scream is the sound of children, which is why children in my village are required to cry out in confirmation of the newborn's arrival. This confirmation satisfies something in the psyche of the newborn, who is now ready to surrender to being present in this world. I have often wondered, what would happen to the newborn if there were no answer? Can infants recover from the damage done to their souls as a result of a message at birth that they are on their own?

Throughout children's life in the village there is a strong message that they belong to a community of people who value them almost beyond anything else. It starts when grandparents participate in the birthing and are the first to hold the newborn. Because the newborn is considered a villager who has just arrived from a long trip that started in the land of the ancestors, the people most recognizable to them are the old ones; grandparents look pretty much like those who were left behind. Another reason for the presence of the elderly is that having just arrived, the newborn shares with the grandparents a close proximity to the Other World. Naturally they bond together.

This relationship between grandparents and children is reenacted periodically and in public while the rest of the village watches. On a sunny afternoon, the village gathers in three distinct groups. The first is the group of elders or grandparents. The second consists of the children and grandchildren. The third group is made up of the remaining villagers, the adults. Grandparents are seated each on a stool in one tight, straight row, dressed in their better clothing, and the children are posted some sixty to ninety feet away. Someone intones a song, and everybody, including the children, sings.

But the kids, as they sing, run toward the row of elders, each one selecting a grandparent and focusing an eye on him or her while singing and running. As the song ends, these children crash into the laps of their chosen grandparent. Some collisions are mild, others are more rough, but the overall impact is sweet and loving. After the crash, the children return to their position and start all over again. Every time a crash results in the fall to the ground of the elder and child, they are out of the game. If, after the third time for boys, or the fourth time for girls, there is no fall, then the child must switch to a different elder.

At first, this ritual play while singing praise to the great mothers and fathers may not be understandable. It is not a competition, yet everybody looks forward to the crash, and everybody is happy whether there is a fall or not. Very rarely does a grandparent fall as a direct result of a grandchild jumping on him or her. The interesting thing is the bonding that it permits, and the fact that it becomes the subject of talk long after it is over. Gradually, children don't distinguish between different grandparents. Every old person comes to be known as Grandpa or Grandma. Reinforcing this idea is the general party that follows the crashing ritual, which the entire village takes part in. Here each child dances with a grandparent while everyone spurs them on with great excitement. The party with the very old and the very young is very exciting to watch.

These examples suggest that what is required for the maintenance and growth of a community is not corporate altruism or a government program, but a villagelike atmosphere that allows people to drop their masks. A sense of community grows where behavior is based on trust and where no one has to hide anything. There are certain human powers that cannot be unleashed without such a supportive atmosphere, powers such as the one that enables us to believe in ancestors and to believe in our ability to unlock potentials in ourselves and others far beyond what is commonly known. When an individual feels connected to an entire community, this connection can extend far beyond the living world. This suggests that a healthy connection with one another will spill over into a connection with the ancestors and with nature. Similarly, the struggle to connect in this world will extend itself to the Other World.

HEALING, ART, AND COMMUNITY

Community can create a container for natural abilities that can find no place in a world defined by economics and consumerism—abilities such as artistic talent or shamanic gifts, healing skills and clairvoyance. These talents are widely recognized in indigenous communities because indigenous people assume that the artist is a priest or a priestess through whom the Other World finds an entrance into this world. If the priest or the priestess regards with reverence and humility the world where his or her art originates, then the work done become lasting and impressive. If not, the artist does not last very long. The artist as an artisan of the sacred can cooperate in bringing the sacred to birth in this world. Indigenous people believe that without artists, the tribal psyche would wither into death.

Carvers and painters produce their things for ritual purposes, which are enjoyed by the entire village. Storytellers act like the repository of the village genealogical memory.

Artistic ability, the capacity to heal, and the vision to see into the Other World are connected for indigenous people. In my village there is only a thin line between the artist and the healer. In fact, there is no word in the Dagara language for art. The closest term to it would be the same word as sacred. It is as if there is an intrinsic sacredness to artistic symbolism. This is perhaps why art objects do not go on show. This is also perhaps why the artist does not think about how to gain public stature. In the village the ability to birth art is a sign of approval by the Spirit World.

The blessed nature of the artist commands respect and reverence from everyone. The art that results from such a blessed hand is in turn approached with fear, reverence, and respect because it is accepted as a shipment straight from the Other World. The artist through whom the delivery is made is regarded with awe and approached as the carrier of a gateway. It is as if he or she is a doorway to the other side. More often than not, the artist is not observed while at work. When busy, he or she is occupied by Spirit. No one should disturb a person who is consulting with Spirit, or he may attract the Spirit's wrath.

The connection between the artist as a sacred healer and the community is undeniable. To produce beauty consistently requires a healthy community. Therefore the artist is the pulse of the community; his or her creativity says something about the health of the community. This is because another role of the artist consists in acting as the spiritual fountain of the community. The beauty artists produce quenches the thirst of the village. Sometimes I have wished that there were a museum of art in my village. But then I remember that collecting art objects in one place, to indigenous people, would be a sign that people want something from the Other World that is not being supplied adequately; they would be experiencing a thirst that is not being quenched. And, even more important, it would mean that the community is in struggle, is experiencing a longing for the sacred. In such a place of struggle, the longing for the sacred is so enhanced that people are collecting and storing art objects. From an indigenous point of view, the isolation of self and community from Spirit appears to have translated into the imprisonment of art. The museums of the West, from an indigenous perspective, speak poignantly of the sharply felt longing for Spirit experienced by modern people.

SPIRITUAL CRISIS AND COMMUNITY

In African indigenous culture, just as there is high respect for artists and healers, there is a similar respect for the person who is experiencing a psychological crisis. This crisis is seen as the result of an intense interaction with the Other World, making the person think and act crazily. Resolving that crisis, in an indigenous community, results in releasing that person's gifts to the community—the very gifts won through the person's intense dealings with Spirit. Every time I encounter a modern person who is in crisis, a person whom other people refer to as crazy, I wonder what gifts are being lost to the community.

Countless people wake up in the middle of the night wondering what is going on around and within them. Some think they are crazy, some feel something incredible is happening to them, and others just go insane. This problem is not specific to the modern world, it happens also in Africa. The difference is that in the modern world, errant behavior in a person is regarded as a personal problem, concerning only that individual. The possibility that there is a larger meaning to be found in the person's experiences, which might translate into something meaningful for that person's community, is rarely considered.

A story from my village illustrates the gifts that can be released to the community if a psychological crisis is resolved through the attention of the whole community. Every time I have gone home to my village over the past three years, there was a young hunter who would delight in bringing me game from the wild. The young man never came home empty-handed after a night-long hunting spree. For each of the days I was in the village, he would present me with a wide variety of wild meat. It so happened that one week he disappeared for three days and three nights. No one could tell why he hadn't come back. On the third day, the entire village decided to suspend everything else and go looking for the hunter who didn't return.

Past experience had taught everyone of the rather mystical aspect of the hunter, so they considered him vulnerable to becoming the hunted. It had been a few generations since a hunter had disappeared. Everyone was concerned because no one could recall ever escorting a lost hunter back to the village alive; the villagers always discovered either that the hunter had been hunted down by a spirit that lured him to his hiding place by masquerading as an animal, or that the hunter had hit some sort of sudden energy surge in the wilderness and had been absorbed by it. This is known in divination. Either way, a hunter that didn't report home was always feared to be lost to the village forever.

When the village decided to stop normal activity that day and go look for the hunter, the dead silence of the people was reminiscent of an imminent funeral ritual. Two-thirds of the village disappeared into the bush following the hunter's trail. At dusk, they heard a man singing and screaming. It was the village hunter. He had been jumped by a spirit. He was naked, with no weapon in his hands. He was full of heat, and his spirit was on fire. When he noticed the crowd of human beings coming toward him, he dashed off in terror. People tried to reassure him that they were not his enemy, but he would not listen. A race ensued, which, as dusk was yielding to the dark of night, was becoming dangerous.

The crowd eventually caught him, tied him up, and brought him back to the village. The priest of the earth shrine consulted with the diviners and confirmed that the hunter had been jumped by a spirit. The spirit explained that for years it had anonymously followed and helped him in his hunting. The hunter had been ungrateful, never recognizing that his success was not luck but the result of the spirit's friendly presence in the wild around him. Had the hunter consulted with the diviner earlier, he would have been told that it was time to put up a shrine for the spirit that hunted with him at night that had brought him good results. But since the hunter had not done this, the spirit had no choice but to make itself known in a dramatic way. It had decided that the hunter would know no sense of direction, and would recognize no one in his own village, until a shrine was set up for the spirit guide and a gift of a white chicken brought to it.

Of course the shrine was set up at once and the sacrifice performed, along with other rituals that are customary in these circumstances. The next morning, the young hunter awoke in shame at finding out that he was naked. (Nakedness has almost disappeared in my village due to the import of affordable used clothing from the United States.) He was told the story of his behavior when the village found him, and he told the village about how he was jumped by his own spirit guide. Without the village, and without the community's ability to consult Spirit for guidance, what would have happened to this young hunter?

A community must look inside itself and its members for instances of powerful spiritual connection. This not only guarantees ongoing attention to one another and diminishes our vulnerability to anonymity, but also softens the pains associated with spiritual awakening

For its own benefit and that of its members, the community must provide a way to support people undergoing crises resulting from the activity of Spirit. The community supports the person through ritual. Such people often experience great agitation and may act inappropriately because they are a vessel of Spirit. A ritual for assisting a person experiencing a spiritual awakening would involve placing the individual at the center of the village's attention; this attention settles the person's agitation. Without a ritual structure, people undergoing a natural emergence of Spirit within often feel as if they are going crazy or are imagining things. As long as Spirit is determined to disturb them, they will display unavoidable symptoms. Once this kind of awakening begins, it is psychologically and emotionally damaging to be unable to integrate one's life. Community provides the safety net in which an individual can rest until he or she has become reintegrated.

Why this safety net? Because, as explained earlier in the context of childbirth, the attention of the entire village to one person is motivated by the conviction that each person is the carrier of something that the village desires. The proof of this is in the fact of birth itself. A person's coming into this world testifies to the fact that one is a giver. And so everyone's behavior toward everyone else is based on the encouragement to develop each person's gift.

In an indigenous community, each person is precious. No one is born on this earth without a reason, a special purpose. Failure or inability to perform one's function in the village places a person in a constant state of crisis. So crises from either of these two sources—the embodiment of a new spirit wanting to emerge, and the impossibility of doing what one came into the village to do—must be addressed by the community.

In the chapters that follow, we look at two sets of relationships that are vital to a community: mentors working with youth, and elders who safeguard the health of the community. Both mentors and elders assist individuals in remembering and claiming their purpose in life. Rituals of healing, which also increase awareness in the individual and the community, will be addressed in parts three and four.

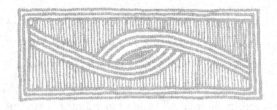

5.

Mentors and the Life of Youth

Avoid three kinds of Master:
Those who esteem only themselves,
For their self-esteem is blindness;
Those who esteem only innovations,
For their opinions are aimless, without meaning;
Those who esteem only what is established;
Their minds are little cells of ice.

—THOMAS MERTON,
"Readings from Ibn Abbad"

There are certain things without which young people cannot survive and flourish, and mentoring is one of them. Westerners see adolescents as fundamentally naive about life. By contrast, the tribal mentor sees a youth as someone who already contains all of the knowledge that he or she needs, but who must work with an older, more experienced person to "remember" what they know. A mentor therefore is not a teacher in the strict sense of the term, but a guide who shows the way, working from a position of respect and affinity, addressing the knowledge within the young person. The pupil is not an ignorant person in the eye of his or her mentor. The pupil is seen as a storehouse, a repository of something the mentor is quite familiar with and very interested in, something the mentor himself has and knows very well. The mentor perceives a presence knocking at a door within the pupil, and accepts the task of finding, or becoming, the key that opens the door. There develops a relationship of trust between mentor and pupil, motivated by love, and without which success would be unlikely.

AWAKENING GENIUS

Mentoring is aimed at increasing security, clarity, and maturity in the young person. It seeks to develop the genius within a young person so that the youth can arrive at his or her destination—the sharing of one's gifts within the community. In Greek mythology, for example, Athena plays the role of a mentor in showing Odysseus how to proceed home safely from Troy and in protecting Odysseus' young son, Telemachus, on his journey in search of his father. The maturation that follows shows that young Telemachus wants to grow. Similarly, in Africa, the journey of a young person through adolescence is taken with the help of a mentor, so that the young person may grow into the mature adult who can live out his or her purpose in the community, giving of one's own genius and receiving, in turn, the help of others.

At the core of mentoring is the understanding that genius must be invited out of a person. People carry to this world something important that they must deliver, and mentors help to deliver that genius to the community. To see the genius in a young person is to give it the fertile ground required for it to burst forth and blossom, for it is not enough to be born into this world loaded with such a beauty. The newborn must be assisted in giving birth to the genius that he is born with. Failure to do so kills that genius along with the person carrying it. The community responsible for the death of an inner genius is like an assassin. The community that is able to receive the person's genius gives birth to the adult who is able to contribute his or her healing gifts to that community.

The West defines genius as a great intelligence, or an exceptional talent. I don't reject that definition. But it is different from the indigenous definition, which sees genius as an open line that flows through a person from the Other World. It seems to me that limiting the meaning of *genius* to intelligence or talent displaces it from its real source and privatizes it in the individual. If genius has no grounding in the sacred, then it becomes easy for the community to ignore it if it chooses. In the traditional context, the community does not have a choice. The community is obligated to awaken the newcomer's genius, and the ritual welcoming of the newborn into this world is the community's official acceptance of this responsibility.

If genius is the expression of the sacred in an individual, then the individual's link to the Other World is the spiritual umbilical cord that cannot be cut until its owner is fully awakened into his gift. Just as our umbilical cord cannot be cut until we are fully in this side of reality, we must nurture and maintain the genius until its complete birth in this world. To cut outright is to kill.

I stress the role of community because a mentor distinct from a community is very hard to conceive of in the indigenous mind. The point is that there is no use delivering something to a destination where there is nobody to receive it. The very purpose of mentoring is twofold. One is to recognize and awaken; the other is to facilitate the delivery of the genius to the community. In a culture where community matters more than anything, mentoring becomes an essential social responsibility. People assume that a mentor will come forward who is appropriate for the particular youth in question.

Because genius is sacred, originating not in this world but another, it must be approached ritualistically, that is, symbolically—with respect and even reverence. Though we will discuss the subject of ritual in depth later in this book, it is useful to point out now that genius understands the language of ritual better than any other language. Through ritual, genius feels invited to come out into this world. Ritual makes the host of genius feel recognized, because ritual shows that the people inviting genius to come forth do speak its language and therefore must mean well. Making the host feel welcome and recognized is necessary because the birth of genius is an intense emotional event in which the pupil is vulnerable. Indigenous people tend to approach emotion, and sometimes even pain, as a sacred thing because they think it means that something in the person is moving out in order to let something else come in. The tension between the incoming and outgoing energies produces pain. So the pain involved in bringing genius to birth evokes ritual. The stretching of the body's physiology out of its normal parameters, which is what allows the shift to happen, is supported through ritual, as a serious and sacred thing.

MENTORING IN THE VILLAGE

In the village, the awakening of dormant knowledge can be extremely dangerous to the person who carries it. I knew a young girl who, at the age of thirteen, became aware of something in herself—the ability to see events in people's lives before they happened, especially harmful things. There was a frightening clarity to these events, and she was unable to contain them and be calm when they appeared to her. When she was in public, it was not infrequent to hear her suddenly scream after looking at someone for a short time. It was as if an upcoming event in the person's life was staring back at her, putting her into a visionary state for a brief moment. She would then run to her companions and cling to them, protesting that she did not want to see what she had seen. Sometimes events would appear to her even if the persons involved were not present.

Her description never included anything extraordinary from the Other World. She merely saw illnesses present in people or evil tendencies about to become manifest in others.

People in the village began to worry about her. On the one hand, traditional customs require that the person in whom knowledge has awakened must first be put under close observation. It is as if a premature intervention would result in incomplete processing of the awakened knowledge and could therefore lead to dementia. But watching the young girl was hard. Every event she saw affected her profoundly. For the next few days or weeks, she was so shaken that she could not even move by herself. Basically each vision was a crisis, like the eruption of a fever, since her body was oven hot for hours after the experience. There came a time when she did not want to go out for fear of seeing something strange. The simple thought of going for a walk threw her into delirium.

It was then that an old woman was introduced to her. After working closely with this woman for one year as her mentor, the girl was able to divine and to predict what would happen to other people with great clarity and accuracy. I do not know in detail how the old woman helped the young girl develop and control her abilities, for the details of the mentoring relationship remain strictly between the two people involved. All I know is that the girl had to bathe herself in an herb solution for weeks and sit by the side of her mentor as she practiced her craft. They would spend many long hours together discussing the subject of their common expertise, until the young girl began to feel comfortable with her abilities.

The example above suggests that the psyche and spirit of a person develop at a faster pace during adolescence than at any other time. Hence the need for someone to support the young person at this critical juncture. The mentor is not a teacher but rather a mirror. The mentor sees in the young one's struggle what he or she has been able to overcome. The pupil sees in the mentor the destination of his or her own journey, and there is a unique reciprocity in their relationship. The mentor focuses on the character and/or spirit of the young person and seeks to bring that person's unique gifts to full fruition within the community. The mentor is, in a sense, the midwife of the adolescent's spirit.

I have heard many stories from Westerners that are not unlike this young girl's story. Psychospiritual crises affect Western as well as indigenous youth. Mentoring is a model that can address the crises of Western as well as indigenous youth, for in a mentoring model the young person is regarded as an asset to the community, a gift in the process of being delivered to the whole village. The village waited with patience while the girl suffered from her gift, rather than judge her as spiritually or emotionally unbalanced. People's patience was motivated by their desire not only to know what genius she carried, but their desire also for wisdom in determining who should mentor her. In this little girl's case, her special talent is called *gniéru*, that is, "a widened eyesight."

I learned how to awaken the art of divination that lay within me through working side by side with my mentor, or as we call it in the village, my *madaba*. At first when my mentor came to me, I had no clue about what was happening. I initially thought Uncle Guisso was simply examining me, since every young person must be examined by a clairvoyant for early detection of any malfunction in their psyche. In the traditional examination, the client or patient sits facing the diviner, who then examines his tools—an extensive array of mundane objects, including shells, bones, stones, and metals. While he examines the tools, he extracts from them, in an esoteric or mystical way, information pertinent to the client. Because at the time I had just come out of a formal Western school where teacher and student had a clear-cut relationship—the teacher acting clearly as the authority and the student as the ignorant—I was under the impression that if Guisso was not examining me, then he probably was trying to teach me something.

As he first spoke to me about divination, I wondered what use it could be to me to learn about such rituals. I assumed, along with most other people in my village, that divining was out of the question for someone who knew how to read and write. Diviners were reluctant to examine literate people because they assumed that the literate person would not cooperate with an esoteric prescription, namely a ritual intended to heal a problem. They were also reluctant to work with literate people because it was assumed that certain kinds of knowledge don't mix with others; it was important not to allow two systems so radically opposed to come together because it was feared that the person in whom they mix would not be able to manage them. Literacy represents a kind of clairvoyant knowledge that diviners think does not agree with magical knowledge. Their approach may be a reaction to colonialism, for the brutality perpetrated on indigenous people under colonial rule came from literate people. So it is easy for indigenous diviners to conclude that literacy is a violent knowledge bent on attacking any nonliterate knowledge.

Guisso, however, was not the kind of person willing to enter into debate about what his purposes should be. As I found out later on, people like him simply do what they have to do and leave the discussion for after they finish. This means that nonliterate mentors share or teach by action, not by dissection and instruction. They are reluctant to prove why anything works and do not want to talk about what they practice.

I have a sense that in the West, discussion and debate are very important, especially in the context of education. This is another area where the West differs from the indigenous world. Indigenous people would prefer to preserve in its naked form the material encountered in one's experience. Experience, to indigenous people, looks like a different kind of discourse that parallels, but does not intersect, the verbal. The more intense an experience, the more likely indigenous people are to leave it in the language in which it came rather than to discuss and dissect it with words. It is almost as if discussing diminishes what is being discussed. Villagers feel that words conquer experience, dislodging experience from its rightful place of power. So unless powerful experiences and ideas are addressed poetically, or with proverbs, people don't want to take the risk of losing in a fog of words what they have struggled so hard to acquire.

Day after day, I would sit next to Guisso, the diviner, while he consulted with people, interpreting the situations of each person by using symbols as a writing in a traditional and mystical language. This language was encoded in cowrie shells, old bones, worn-out pieces of metal, stones of different sizes and shapes. Once in a while he would ask for my help, pointing to a symbol of divination and pretending he did not have a full grasp of its meaning. Caught always by surprise, I would mutter something, and in response he would elaborate upon my point, making no contradictory statement. I assumed that the man was usually just being kind, although sometimes, in looking steadily at the symbolism, I could logically trace and translate circumstances even though I had to convince myself that I was not making things up.

I remember, for example, this woman who brought her sick daughter for divination. Guisso looked at his reading materials, picked up a little stone and a piece of metal, and put them on the side. Then he looked again for a while and asked me to pick something. My attention was on a little talisman that sat in the middle of a V-shaped piece of wood. Guisso said, "Therefore the medicine should be a pearl to hang on the child's ankle, right?" I did not know what to say, but I must have said yes. Guisso went on to explain that the stone that appeared was a symbol of the child's connection with an ancestor who is her protector. The symbol of the ancestor had to be worn by the child or she wouldn't survive. He put the stone down and picked up the piece of metal in his hand, explaining that this was the link. "What link?" I asked. "The link between the child and her protector in the world of the ancestors." I wanted to ask why or how, but I checked myself. I knew he would not answer.

The real challenge came when he would suspend a reading process midway and ask me to take over because he had to attend to something else. I saw myself mechanically executing his order, cloaked with a terrifying feeling of failure as I embarked on this random journey to fish out information from this utterly bizarre book. I never remembered how I carried on from where he left off, nor did he ask me how it went when he returned long after the end of the session. I may have become used to doing it alone without being reprimanded for mistakes or scolded for indulging in false statements. Whatever happened, I became gradually aware that I knew what he knew, and that his role with me was not based on the fact that he was my uncle but my mentor.

Mentoring is a role that is assumed not strictly by age, but by ability and experience. Guisso is an old man in his seventies, an elder by Dagara standards. But more parents than grandparents are mentors. It is not surprising to find mentors aged twenty-five to thirty years if the need and the knowledge are present. Similarly the people mentored cover a wide range of ages, but almost always the pupil is younger than the mentor, if not by age, at least with respect to the knowledge being exchanged in that relationship. This is because in indigenous Africa, knowing means becoming old. To say that someone is old is to say that this person knows something, or has experienced something valuable. Furthermore, the mature self is hardened in the field of experience by awareness. In contrast, the word *young* refers not just to age but also to the absence of awareness.

The way villages are structured leaves no room for a young person to escape having a mentor. The cohesiveness and identity of a village require this kind of caretaking. Unlike loosely formed modern communities, where each person is often preoccupied by his or her own affairs, village life requires that most things be done collectively because people are very tightly connected. Tight connection fosters friction. In turn, friction among people deepens their sense of belonging. People bound by community are sure, at some point, to get on one another's nerves. This is not considered a bad thing, but rather a part of the natural human experience.

CONFLICT WITH MENTORS

Some mentoring relationships encounter the heat of conflict and the chaos of discord. It is as if the birthing of the knowing self must undergo tremors and shakes designed to remove the layers of protection under which the gold of knowledge hides. This is why they say in the village that an unruly youth is asking in his own way for someone to guide him.

My father's story of his relationship with his mentor illustrates the conflict that may arise in a mentoring relationship. My father told me that prior to and after his initiation it was almost impossible to maintain a reasonable communication with the man in charge of him. He describes his experience as a loving rebellion that he tried in vain to avoid until he was in his midtwenties. It seemed as if part of his love could be expressed only in terms opposite love. He would fail to show up at his mentor's home or would show up at a time other than agreed upon and feel extreme angry heat bursting through him as he witnessed his mentor ignoring him. One day, my father confessed, he was so unruly that his mentor finally spoke out to discipline him. This led to a short but open verbal altercation, which ended with his breaking into tears in his mentor's arms, screaming insults at him, yet staying gently in his arms.

"I loved to get mad when I was young," said my father, "and Guiliko, my mentor, had plenty of ways to satisfy my fire. He would ask me to sit in the sun and wait for him while he made some offerings at different altars in the house. I thought this meant that he would come out quickly. But he didn't, so I would go wait under the shade of the tree. When he came out and saw me resting under the tree, he would yell at me and tell me I was lazy. What's lazy about waiting? Who wouldn't get angry for this? This is how easy it was for Guiliko to make people angry.

"All I needed was for him to teach me his carving. He was the best. He had me cutting trees for a year before I was allowed even to sit and watch him do the carving. Then it took another long time before he allowed me to touch his carving tools."

My father said he burned from within so badly that he needed a little conflict to flush out some of the fire in him. His mentor was the right person, because every time my father received no thanks from him for doing something right, it made him want to kill him. "I knew I was a good carver after three years with him, but he waited another two years before acknowledging that. That day, I was so pissed that I cried in his arms while telling him how bad he was with people and particularly with me. But I loved him."

This is a story I could relate to because in the course of my own relationship with my mentor I remember more vividly the times when I yearned to kill him than the times when I wanted him alive for my own sake. Almost every time I was with him, something he did or said, something he did not do or failed to say, irritated me profoundly and stole a few curses out of my mouth. I must confess that though he is still alive, I can't stand seeing him because our conversation is almost always a slippery journey into the sticky mud of disappointment. Yet I love my mentor beyond what I can say. I must say here that a mentor in the village never tells the student when he or she is finished, because this is not the mentor's responsibility. The student is supposed to know when he or she is finished, and the mentor must acknowledge that and give the student a blessing. This seldom happens smoothly or beautifully. I don't remember how I parted with my mentor, but I know it was not ceremonial. I think I just quit, not because I had learned enough, but because I was tired of him. We had chosen each other to do the things that we did, but our personalities were quite different, and it was up to me to recognize when the usefulness of our working together had come to an end.

MENTORS AND PARENTS

Since in the village mentors play some of the roles that in the West are assumed by parents, I need to spend some time clarifying the different roles as villagers see them. Most villagers believe that the disciplining of children is better done by others than by the biological parents, since in the village parents often resort to spanking and verbal ferocity. These methods tell children quickly that they are out of line and may quiet them down for a while. But another result is that the children come to prefer being parented by other fathers and mothers of the village, including their mentor.

In the village it is acceptable for children to say that they love another mother or father better than their biological parent, since everyone who has children is considered a parent to every child in the village. In fact, it is normal for children to choose favorite "parents of the day" on a regular basis. A child will pick an adult whom she or he loves and spend the whole day with that adult. My sister, who has several children, says laughingly that she sometimes has to bribe her children to spend the day with her. The result is that children may get more attention from all the mothers and fathers of the village than from their own. This does not imply that parents enjoy caring for other people's children more than their own. It just means that their biological parents are not always on top of the children's lists. Consequently, if you hear someone in the village call a person father or mother, do not assume that this is the biological father or mother. It may be an aunt or uncle or other adult with whom the person spent a lot of time in their childhood. It also may be just another adult in the village who, by reason of having children, was considered a father or mother to every child in the village.

If mentors are spiritual parents, biological parents are stepping-stones, the points of departure for children. At their best, biological mothers and fathers are friends of their children. They can help their children as special friends do in times of need. But their limitation is to be almost helpless in the business of bringing out the child's true spirit. This is where the mentor enters in, since his or her spirit becomes for the child a mirror of what the child is feeling inside. Consequently, their relationship has some content that is based on Spirit, in contrast to the parental relationship, which is based on biology. The latter relationship is fixed and cannot be changed, which sometimes makes it a source of irritation, especially on the subject of discipline, because the child is prone to see discipline as punishment. In contrast, the relationship with a mentor can be changed, which makes choice more apparent.

LOCATION OF THE MENTOR

Although living in the same area does not prohibit a mentoring relationship, it is common among the indigenous that the mentor and the pupil live in different villages. This is in part because the pupil's receptivity increases by leaving his or her familiar environment. A little psychological distance is considered good for the growth of the pupil. It forces attention and respect when the mentor is somewhat far away. You can't walk five miles to spend the day in a state of distraction and disrespect. If the mentor is some distance away, it indicates that the constant physical presence of the mentor is not necessary. The real issue is quality of time rather than quantity.

For example, a while ago I heard that my young sister had become the vessel of a powerful genius awakening in her. In village language, the genius in her was being supported and fed from the Other World by a pair of tiny little beings similar to what Western mythology refers to as leprechauns. The *kontombli* were well meaning, but my sister's young frame was not at the time suited for the intensity involved in interacting with these beings. For months her body was thinning out under the huge pressure of shock waves from the presence of these beings. She told me that there came a time when she could no longer go to sleep at night because of what would happen. As soon as she closed her eyes, she would reopen them, only to notice that the pitch dark had been replaced with a bright light. Then from above, and with a fuzzy sound, would come a being illuminated by yellow light. The little being would present her with a cup full of an unknown potion, and a bag full of cash. Then he would say to her that this was her medicine.

Sometimes she would be ordered in the middle of the night to go see a healer in a remote village. She would get up and begin walking fearlessly along the dark narrow trail of the tribe toward the village. Her consultation with the shaman always resulted in a confirmation of what was hap-

pening to her—she was privileged to have beings from the Other World
elect to work with her. My sister, on the other hand, wanted to reject the
process, saying that she was not worthy and that someone else in the family should be the one to be linked with these beings.

The village found her a female mentor from a different tribe located
one hundred miles away. She moved to that tribe and began learning how
to identify the kinds of herbal medicines necessary to help connect herself
with these beings. Indeed, when one is in this kind of situation, the only
way to end the turmoil is to find the proper medicine to open and clear the
channel so that one can hear, see, and feel the Other World loud and clear,
not merely in a dream state. My sister washed herself with the essences of
the appropriate herb, and on the thirty-sixth day she again saw the *kontombli,* including the world they come from, and learned from them directly how to work with people to better their lives. It took this long
because of the delayed cleansing effect of the herbs. Apparently these
herbs were supposed to wipe out impurities in her aura that stood in the
way of her seeing anything.

The last time I saw her, my sister still had to clear some debris from
her communication channel with these beings. The voices of these beings
when in communication through her with our world were still too difficult
to interpret consistently. I am told that the next time I see her, the voices
of the Other World speaking through my sister will be clearly audible.
She is now one hundred miles away from our village, in the communication headquarters of the *kontombli,* undergoing intensive education under
the disciplined supervision of her mentor.

The emotional bond that develops between the mentor and the pupil
can also benefit from distance. One needs time to process emotional
lessons. Besides, constant presence can become a harmful codependency.
Here in the West, where youth often live on the edge, the danger of emotional codependency is always high when a needy pupil meets a real mentor. Like a husband and wife who can't live apart for any length of time,
or like lovers enthralled with one another, mentor and pupil run the risk
of losing sight of their purpose. In part as a means of reducing the likeli-

hood of an unproductive relationship, mentoring is almost always a relationship between two people of the same gender.

MENTORING IN THE WEST

In the West, mentoring must take as many forms as is allowed by the structure of society, taking into account the pressure of daily life, the radical difference of geography, and more important the rather narrow vision of reality and the complicated notion of the sacred and the supernatural. Mentoring cannot wait for a villagelike context to happen, but it can share, without compromising, the indigenous notion that a genius in someone is about to be born. Therefore the first form mentoring must take is simply recognizing the presence of genius in a young person. It begins with paying careful attention to the young person. The best medicine for a young man in crisis is listening. Listening equals respect and recognition. A young woman, feeling recognized, can begin to develop the trust that is needed for her crisis to be resolved and her inner gifts to be delivered to the world. Recognition begins with supportive attention. Every grown-up who gives supportive attention to a young person can see existing within that youth something that the adult knows, a pattern of behavior that is familiar because the grown-up experienced it in his or her own life. This behavior, which is the symptom of something bigger wanting to burst out, needs attention, and attention is something that anybody, Western or not, can give.

I still remember the effect I produced on the first young boy I worked with in this country when I pointed out to him what was happening in his psyche. This boy, we will call him George, was in serious trouble. He could not stay in school because he found nothing in it worth relating to. His own parents believed that money would resolve everything, only to find out that their teenage son cared very little about their wealth. Every word they uttered to him was suspect, every suggestion a threat. His parents were at a loss about what to do.

George came to me for a divination after hearing me talk at his school about the value of rites of passage and feeling moved. I noticed that he needed, first and foremost, to be confirmed in his visionary abilities, and to be encouraged to pursue the kinds of studies at school that would lead up to his successful involvement with other people. His reaction to my simple observation that he had visionary gifts and that because of that people often thought he was crazy was almost hysterical. I expected him to say something like, "So what?" Instead he burst into tears at being recognized as a seer, a person with great vision and sensitivity. He confided to me things not dissimilar to that which my sister experienced, except that in his case the only mentors he could work with were dead authors like Rumi, Krishnamurti, Nietzsche, and Yogananda. His head was a warehouse of disordered supernatural images clashing with his culture's view. His ability to see things was his genius, and he was aware of it, but it was a gift that immobilized him until someone else stepped forward to acknowledge and accept it .

From then on George was willing to discuss how he could apply his innate ability to enrich his daily life. Months later, when we met again, George was back in school and doing well. He still did not enjoy being there. He wanted an alternate way of education and had decided that I might be it. But he accepted a compromise, which was to stay at school. I remained in touch with George and noticed after two years that the person I first met had given way to a new one. The new George was dedicated to life and to people. He wanted to become a healer in the modern sense of the term. I lost personal contact with him a year and a half later, but I am aware that he is still doing well.

George was not a pupil the way I was toward Guisso. More often than not, George and I would simply discuss the experiences he was having. He was profuse with visions, dream images, and striking coincidences that occurred so often that in the end he did not believe they were coincidences. I quietly listened most of the time, and confirmed his sanity the rest of the time. That was all he needed. We prayed together to Spirit, made shrines, and talked to each other about how good and effective such practice was.

This is one method of mentoring that can work in the modern world. If there is a difference between this and indigenous mentoring, there is also some similarity. In both cases the mentor observes that something is about to come forth from within a young person that needs the direction of someone else to become manifest. It is as if the youth is in labor and in need of a midwife. Any assistance offered needs to rest on the premises that the young person is not insane or misbehaving. It needs to honor the value of the depth of experience going on in the psyche of the other whether or not one understands it completely. By doing so, the psyche in the other registers it as availability or even care. This care that sometimes becomes love plants the seeds of change in the other.

As long as someone is in crisis, mentoring is called for. The violence that cripples so many lives is a tearing consequence of a call for mentoring that has met no answer. Yet to mentor requires some giving of the self, some willingness to compromise in the interest of establishing a progressively healthy psyche and spirit in the other. This includes the willingness to be vulnerable, to learn gently about the world of the other, instead of jumping to conclusions about the plight of the other. And it also requires finding a way into the emotional world that produced the crisis.

The mentor exists, in the West, in the counselor and the therapist. I see therapy as a form of mentoring, in the sense that what people seek in the therapist is a healing from the crisis that blocks their blossoming. So while in an indigenous context the pupil is usually quite young, in the modern world the pupil may be just as old as, or even older than, the mentor. In this case age does not have to play a particularly important role in establishing a useful mentor relationship here in the West. The urgent need for mentoring relationships in the West may mean that it is no longer possible to maintain certain conventions in the relationship that are common in an indigenous context. Even gender conventions lose their rigidity in the modern world because of the short supply of mentors. A large portion of the people coming to me for spiritual help are women. At first it seemed quite embarrassing to me, but eventually it became clear that in these times of scarcity, one is fortunate to chance upon a mentor at all, let alone a mentor of the same gender.

The program known in this country as Big Brothers/Big Sisters may by inspired by the idea of mentoring, though I do not know enough about it to say if it really parallels indigenous experiences of mentoring. What it does accomplish is pairing up young people at the vulnerable age of adolescence with an adult, other than the parents, who can provide some attention that the young person desperately needs.

One thing common in the West is that, because mentors don't simply appear, pupils often have to chase them down because the crisis they feel deep within does not allow them to sit still and wait for the mentor to show up. When they think they have found an acceptable person, they often express their interest in working with that person in terms of desire for a teacher, but the truth is that they are looking for a mentor. In a long and detailed biographical letter they make a strong case for the necessity of help in this matter. It is as if they recognize in the potential teacher an echo of the knowledge that wants to come out of them. They want to tap into a mentor's experience so they can remember their own deepest purpose in life. The legitimacy as well as the intimacy of the request is almost heartbreaking. Because the ultimate business of life consists of remembering why we are here, these people have been feeling the kicking presence of memory deep inside them. Moved by restlessness, they search for a mentor or a teacher. They sense that their society has treated their genius carelessly. So in the West, adults as well as youth feel the need for mentors.

In the West it is customary to pay teachers and mentors for their services, a practice that would be inconceivable in an indigenous village. Mentors, like any other person capable of making a difference in people's lives, must be saved from being approached primarily as commodities. There has to be a way in which the business of opening a person to himself or herself, of opening to the sacred, is not subjected to the influence

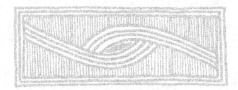

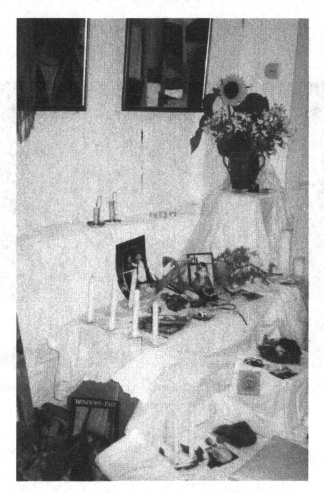

A Western mineral shrine created during a workshop.
White is the predominant color. Photos, books,
and symbolic objects represent remembering and memory,
the primary qualities of the element *mineral*.

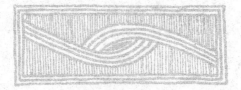

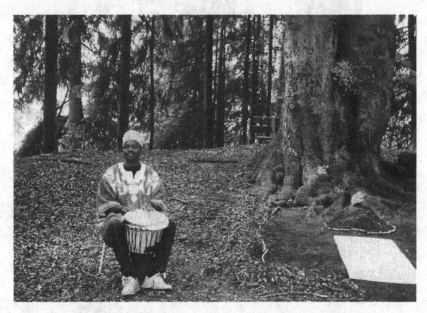

An earth shrine created during a Western workshop. The mound of earth is the simplest symbolic representation of the earth itself.

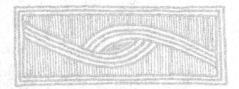

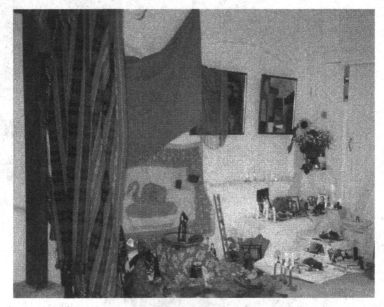

A fire shrine created during a Western workshop. Red is
the predominant color. There are many pictures of relatives and
ancestors, signifying the connection between the element
fire and the world of the ancestors.

A public water shrine
created in the West. In an
urban area, it is a cool refuge
from an otherwise fiery life.

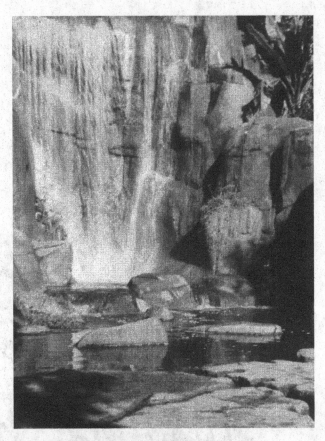

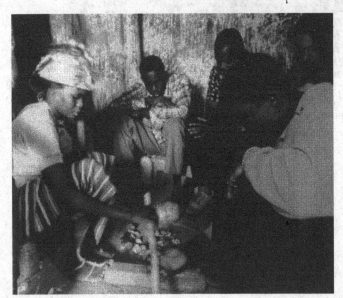

A Dagara diviner
(shaman) in her hut
doing a divination with
a divining stick and
symbolic objects. The
hut is a shrine to the
ancestors, and therefore
a shrine to the element
fire. There is a special
room such as this one
in most of the family
compounds within any
Dagara village.

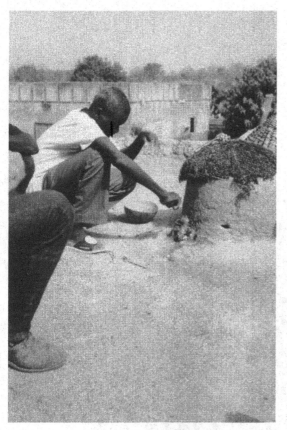

Sitting before a mineral shrine. The shrine is on a roof and is meant to echo the nearby mountains. The symbols of mountain, stone, and mineral are synonymous.

An offering is being made at a nature shrine. The placement of shrines is usually determined through divination, with the intention of locating a shrine at an especially powerful point on the earth.

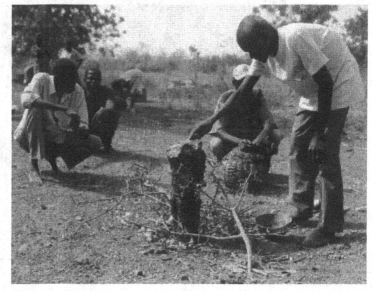

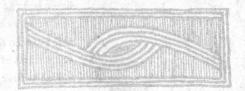

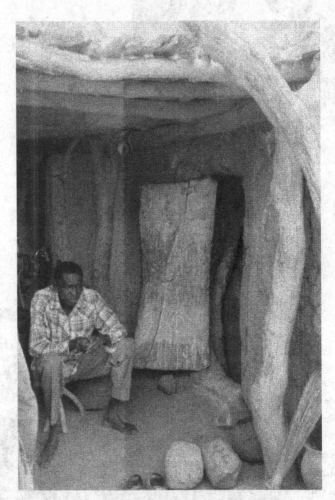

Entrance to the ancestor shrine and working room
of a Dagara diviner and shaman.

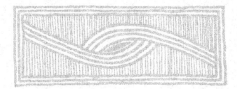

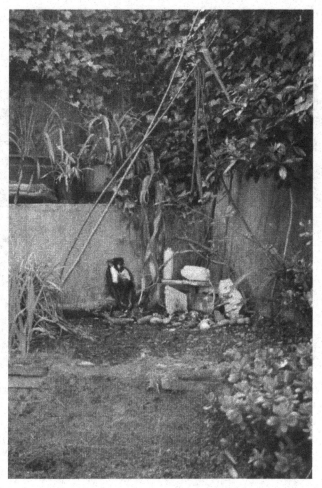

A nature shrine located in the West, sited outdoors and created
with locally found natural objects. This shrine blends
into its surroundings, its purpose being simply to declare
that this is a place to honor the element *nature*
and all it represents.

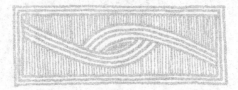

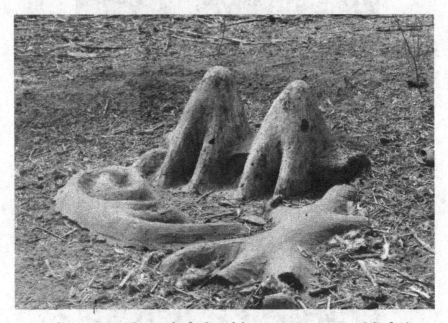

An indigenous water shrine. The fluidity of the swimming creature and the fluidity of the lines of the shrine are representative of the element *water*. Water is the doorway to the Other Worlds inhabited by the non-ancestral spirits, and this shrine sits outside the home and working room of a Dagara diviner.

of money, especially in the context of mentoring. The reason is that something in the economic transaction sends a false message to the psyche that only makes people momentarily feel better.

Does this suggest that consumerism fosters a false view of the relationship between mentor and pupil? On the one hand, it is clear how necessary a mentor is. On the other hand, it is extremely harmful to the mentor and the pupil to establish a relationship that is so flawed from the beginning that it puts both parties at risk. To an indigenous person it would be inconceivable to be a mentor for a living. You become a mentor because your village must live. A mentor cannot be a salesperson or a product for sale. Similarly, a pupil cannot be a client or a customer. A relationship built on these premises would crash as fast as it began.

So the typical modern mentor will be someone who deeply understands his or her pupil from the inside out, one in whom the young person sees the echoes of something she or he is experiencing. This inner resonance in the spirits of the pupil and mentor is more important for establishing a relationship than is the mentor's knowledge of the biographical details of the young person's life—whether the pupil lived in a dysfunctional family or was abused by a drunken father. One becomes a mentor when one is found by a pupil. This is why it is hard to understand the institutionalization of mentorship. You cannot make mentoring your profession because it is the young person who decides whether you are a mentor or not and who requests your services. The greatest mentors don't know they are one till the end. They just try to be as open as possible with their pupil and friend.

So I think that the classical mentoring system known to indigenous people has to be adjusted in the Western context in order to work. If there is a way to view the pupil as a vessel of intensity beneficial to the community, this intensity is worth serving wholeheartedly, since it will lead to everyone's good. For the sake of the future of our children, for the sake of the irreplaceable value of a human being, we need mentors everywhere in the world. Youth anywhere can find in an older person the help capable of bringing forth the genius that wants to be born.

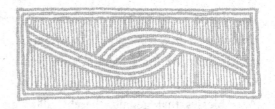

6.

Elders and the Community

gateway of being: open your being, awaken,
learn then to be, begin to carve your face,
develop your elements, and keep your vision
keen to look at my face, as I at yours,
keen to look full at life right through to death,
faces of sea, of bread, of rock, of fountain,
the spring of origin which will dissolve our faces
in the nameless face, existence without face
the inexpressible presence of presences ...
—OCTAVIO PAZ, *The Sunstone*

No matter what culture you belong to, certain personal situations and social relationships are inescapable. For example, common to everyone is the recurrent feeling of needing to expand and to grow. Similarly, you cannot help at certain points in your life feeling the need for the emotional, psychological, and social support of others. Everyone needs to come into some kind of visibility, some sort of recognition. Just as these experiences establish the need for a mentor, they also establish the need for elders. Where a mentor invites the genius of a youth to come out of its hiding, an elder blesses that genius, thereby allowing it to serve efficiently the greater good. We will be talking about two kinds of elders in this chapter, an elder in the formal sense of a village or community leader who helps community members coexist peacefully, and elders in the informal sense of people whose age makes them invaluable resources in community life.

YOUTH AND AGE

In the West, where tremendous energy is invested in the maintenance of youth, to be young means to be vital, attractive, desirable, and at peak performance. Consequently youth has inspired a huge, profitable industry, servicing people's desire for health and for popular images of beauty. While some people peek into mirrors scanning for unwanted residues of age to mask out, others expend tremendous amounts of energy on Nordic Tracks and treadmills covering great distances in the same place. They want to keep in shape, to feel youthful energy, to be strong. Given the commonly held views about youth and age, these efforts are worth the investment.

In African tribal societies in general, and among the Dagara in particular, *young* means "that which is still moist," which needs to be dried and cured in order to last. The young is raw and untested. Its exuberance, beauty, and desirability conceal instability. Its attractiveness is symptomatic of the proximity of the Spirit World. Thus, to indigenous people, desiring youth is tantamount to desiring the Other World. But the presence of the Other World in this world makes it extremely vulnerable. Therefore beauty is synonymous with fragility, and as such needs to be anchored, helped, and granted the right to solidify. When a person embodies natural beauty, this beauty must be enshrined and protected from utter destruction by the forces of evil. The attractiveness of youth, to indigenous people, is first and foremost a call for assistance, the kind of support without which the young cannot blossom into maturity.

The full blossoming out of youth requires taking risks. It demands that one be safe enough to respond to the urge for growth. That safety comes from the hands of older generations. This is where young and old intersect. Here, *old* means someone who is dry, solid, lasting. Thus the old and the elders embody stability, dependability, and wisdom. In this capacity, they become a frame of reference, a resource, a research center.

The wisdom I am trying to point out here for Westerners is obvious. I am trying to say that a retirement house is the wrong place for old people to be. While they are there waiting for their end, the entire society loses a great opportunity: the opportunity to be anchored and thus blessed. The young ones miss having an emotional and even sacred support for doing their work in the world, and the old ones are bored. It is deeply unfortunate if change and progress take place at the expense of elders by robbing them of their legitimate right to connect with their families. To indigenous people, the West's treatment of its elders looks like a production-line view of progress; people become agents of production only, confined eventually to some institution when they can no longer produce.

It appears that in the West, old age is feared because of a loss of powers, but also because it shows our proximity to the Other World, the unknown and the unpredictable. Lack of predictability and control brings into focus the unavoidable frailty of the human condition. Because modern life is characterized by control, old age has become a negative. It is as if by staying young, one can remain distracted enough to forget the painful matter of one's fleeting existence. Where then is the value of progress, if it can't ensure that people in their old age benefit not just from a retirement plan but more importantly from an emotional plan that connects them more deeply to their communities, their children, and grandchildren?

For most traditional African cultures, an elder is one whom the village acknowledges as having reached not only a state of old age but also a state of maturity and wisdom. Elders are repositories of tribal knowledge and life experience, essential resources for the survival of the village, anchoring it firmly to the living foundation of tradition. The old and the elder are the most revered members of the village community and its greatest preservers and nurturers. It is natural that everyone should be attracted by age, to becoming old.

The elder is as important to the community as the newborn, in that they both share a proximity with the Other World, the ancestors' world. The newborn just arrived from there, and the old one, the elder, is preparing to go there. The very young and the very old complement each other because they draw from one another. The very old honor youth as the source of collective physical stability and strength and as recent arrivals to this world, who are more closely connected to the ancestors. Because of the unique relationship of the very young and the very old, among the Dagara, the Lobi, the Fon, and many other communities in West Africa, you will sometimes hear an elder calling a child "Grandpa" or "Grandma." The elder is showing deep respect for the young one, attributing the benefits of age to that young person.

Tradition is the way of the ancestors, the manner in which those who lived before once walked and talked, the knowledge and practices that allowed them to live long enough to bestow life upon others. In indigenous cultures, this is crucial to life, because to forget the way life used to be lived is to become endangered. In my village, for example, there is a very practical, intrinsic belief that in earlier times everything was good, and that everything will remain so as long as ancient ways are allowed to survive in everyday life. Things have changed as a result of Western encroachment. At the core of these changes is a distancing from the past and a fascination with the future. Many people who are taught modern ways have embraced these ways fully and completely except that they could not change the color of their skins. Postcolonial Africa is full of what critics call the acculturated.

But in the traditional view, to look to the old ways is to avoid death. The argument is that our ancestors lived thousands of years under conditions that today would be considered extremely harsh and unbearable. In honor of their wisdom, we feel a sacred approach to, and reverence for, tradition, even when its dictates are not fully understood. The origin of and the need for myth are rooted in this because it provides a worldview, a series of customs that are useful in defining the identity of a society. People don't read the Brothers Grimm, the *Arabian Nights*, or the *Nibelungen* in order to collect evidence of how backward or irrelevant these stories are to the present. They read them because these stories feed something deep in them—evidence that the past is far from obsolete.

Perhaps the respect owed to the elder derives from the perception that the elder is at this critical junction where the natural meets the supernatural and where the ancestors and the divine intersect with the humans. In indigenous African context, this is a place of great freedom and great responsibility. In effect, the elder is almost the only one in the village who can have things his way. But more important, the elder's posture is rooted in his intimate connection to the balance between this life and the Other World, without which village life is a nightmare. Dagara people have made up their minds that they can't live without elders. They know well enough that in the absence of the elders, the container of cultural wholeness breaks and social chaos arises. Indigenous belief in this is so strong that tribal communities cannot understand how cultures can thrive without elders, the same way that a modern person would have a hard time imagining a life without electricity and running water.

PROFILE OF AN ELDER

The profile of an elder includes certain types of behavior and language that are quite visible and strictly followed. This is because age is related to powers that can become lethal when in hands other than those of the old and wise. Among these is the power of blessing. I have become very fond of the elders' words of blessing. Every time I reach the end of my stay in the village, they are the sweetest phrases for me to hear. "May all the ancestors of the tribe accompany you. May they pour vision, insight into your soul. This way you will see through them, feel through them." "We must shower you with the grace of Spirit. May you go with your pocket heavy with precious stones of blessings." I know that what the old wish well is certain to be well in the long run.

At the opposite end of blessing is cursing. "There will be holes every time your foot touches the ground, and a rock will eat your toenails before your feet carry them into the hole. Beware, traveler, the evil forces will notice you more than the forces of fortune. The lion of misfortune will prepare you for dinner as you step out of this place. The sight of your eyes is already folded up and rendered useless. The moment of your perdition has arrived." Thus, what the old do not wish well eventually collapses. Just as the elders' blessing indicates success, the elders' curse invites a misfortune that is very draining to oppose. This is the lethal side of the elders' power, although it is almost never used.

Whatever an elder says, forces in both worlds labor hard to make it happen. A person with this kind of power is naturally revered, feared, and respected, and as a result there are things he can and cannot do or say. For example, under no conditions will elders be heard to shout. This would imply that they have been surprised by something. It would mean also that they are still subject to the unexpected, and that is not characteristic of an elder. An elder cannot indulge in such common social pleasures as drinking alcohol and being drunk. This would imply that there is still a part in them that is moist and searching for growth and expansion. An elder cannot be found in places where motion is fast and excited. These are places for youth. In truth, the position of elder is so awesome that the line between elder and sacred is very thin.

Mastering the powers of an elder is a process that takes place slowly over years at the harsh school of life where the storms of trials and tribulations, of pain and suffering solidify and make sacred the mind, body, and soul of the person. When a person like this speaks, it is as if the Other World is speaking. The pull to listen is natural to one who is familiar with the sound of Spirit. This is also why elders are more accountable than anyone else in the village. But this accountability is even greater in the Other World than in this world because every day brings the elder closer to the world of the Spirit and thus more distant from this world, hence this sense of increased sacredness associated with the voice of an elder. The pull to the Other World also explains the gradual distaste an elder develops for involvement in the ordinary world.

The gender of the elder is important in maintaining the stability of a social community. Female elders, though they have the same qualities as male elders, are often more in demand because of their role as containers and reconcilers. In the village, everyone knows that a female elder is less likely to curse than a male elder. Moreover, it takes a female elder to undo a curse inflicted on someone by a male elder. No one can undo the curse of a female elder. If two people are involved in an argument and a female elder shows up, they will stop before being ordered to do so.

DUTIES OF ELDERS

Elders, like the ancestors, are expected to identify and address what is not working in the village, not to give compliments and praise behavior. In this, they share with mentors the job of executing tasks forwarded to them by the ancestors. In the previous chapter we presented the mentor as a person responsible for inviting the genius out of a person. Once this genius is released, it requires maintenance, sustenance, and growth. This is where the job of the elder begins. The elder holds the space within which this gift operates and encourages it with blessings and with silent nods. Therefore the mentor complements the elder, and to some degree without both, the genius that is coming to birth in the community would have a hard time facing the storms of life.

Thus elders do not express energy, they hold it. When they speak, everybody listens. They often don't speak directly to the person whose situation they are addressing. They don't even name the person. They speak in general terms, but the village knows to whom they refer. For example, when my grandfather watched people overeating, he would say something like, "When someone eats too much, they are sure to experience great pain when they come to initiation." Food is not readily available in indigenous Africa. There are no supermarkets or restaurants. Being hungry is common, and overeating or sometimes even eating enough is seen as destructive to the community.

Elders are also involved in the righting of wrongs, for instance the breaking of an ancestral law. In the culture of the Mossi, the Dogon, the Lobi, the Katsena, the Bobo and others, when someone does something wrong, it is ultimately the ancestors that they offend. For example, when a child acts disrespectfully to his parents, this child is showing disrespect to the ancestors. Eventually, children will have to make their misdeeds right with the ancestors before anything else can go forward. It is like paying a fine. It takes the form of an offering at the altar of the ancestors after confessing one's evildoing. Saying one is wrong and sorry cleans the path for the offering to work.

An elder who witnesses an offense against authority, for instance the ancestors, will first talk about it in general terms in order to draw the person who did it forward to begin reparation, even though his name has not been mentioned. The elder would say something like, "I wonder why someone would deliberately want to put himself in increasing debt." The reason for this indirectness is linked to a rather peculiar understanding of shame and the effect of shaming.

Shame is seen in Dagara culture as a collapsing emotional force that paralyzes the self, and therefore, like grief, shame should be experienced only in a sacred, ceremonial context. In the context of ritual and sacred space, the repentant "sinner" is said to be more capable of deep humility than in an ordinary context. When suffered in daily life, shame compresses the psyche dangerously. The result is that one experiences crippling rejection and ostracism as one's self-esteem is almost exterminated. In Dagara context, this is comparable to death. Shame, like grief, is a powerful emotion. But unlike grief, which emanates from loss, shame arises from a sense of guilt, embarrassment, unworthiness, and disgrace. Shaming is counterproductive. A person in power and responsibility who uses it exposes himself and the other to danger. Distrust, suspicion, and discord are the offspring of shame and attacks against self-esteem. Therefore shaming someone as a way of making that person accountable without the sacred endangers the whole community. The heaviness of the shamed person will in the long run and in subtle ways affect everyone and everything.

In order to heal these embarrassments, one must reexperience them within the context of ritual in order to prevent them from destroying self-esteem and dangerously affecting the community. When an indigenous elder speaks about a shameful act indirectly, no individual feels singled out; all can participate in recognizing that they have done something shameful. There is no public shaming, strictly speaking, but there is a threat of shame if the person does not act immediately by seeking the help of an elder or a healer in order to begin making amends.

Accountability in the form of punishment is debilitating; it encourages concealment, secrecy, and even distortion of reality. It is no wonder that people who are threatened with shaming punishment will try to conceal their deed. Such an urge, to indigenous people, would be legitimate, for it would show a desire to protect the self from annihilation. Accountability defined as a deepening of relationship, by contrast, becomes a productive example in service of the greater whole. For example, when someone causes hurt in someone else, correction rather than punishment is in order; the wrongdoer makes things right by deepening the relationship with the person hurt, maintaining it for the rest of one's life.

ADDRESSING WRONGDOING

Doing wrong is human, and it is with the ancestors, who never forget, that humans must make things right. In this process elders play a mediating role. It is as if they are the ancestral ear in the village, guiding oblivious wrongdoers to act in a healing manner toward themselves and others.

In the village, they say that a person cannot remain right for more than five days. If therefore you have not made a sacrifice to the ancestors of some kind in the past five days, it suggests that your relationship to the ancestors may not be as clear as it was five days before. To some extent, it's like the Catholic confession, which is expected to happen every week before Mass. I remember in the seminary, it was a sin not to appear at confession on Friday evening. People would look at you as if you had not taken a bath for a whole week. In the indigenous village some sacrifice at the altar of the ancestors must be offered. The sacrifice is given to the ancestors so that the negative energy wrapped around a person can be cleansed. The sacrifice must be serious enough to establish the feeling that a burden has been removed and that the individual is committed to refraining from wrongdoing in the future.

When a person does not sacrifice, it affects their family, their children, and the children of their children. This is not unlike some modern fundamentalist belief in the idea of damnation. When a villager has not made a sacrifice, it will come up in the oracles that someone in their house is not doing things right. The head of the family will discreetly try to find out who that person is, often through a diviner or a shaman following the process described in the earlier chapter. Once the wrongdoer is identified, the head of the family will then order him or her into a ritual space in the presence of an elder where there is no shame in admitting out loud what went wrong and then taking the necessary steps to set things right with the ancestors. The presence and nonjudgmental intervention of elders make possible this ritual cleansing.

Very few people can get away with wrongdoing over a lifetime. Dagara believe that unresolved errors are passed on to surviving relatives. This is why tradition ensures that people of every generation fulfill their duties toward the Other World and leave nothing behind undone. For example, there is a story that says that once upon a time a young Dagara man wandered out of the village to hunt. He ran into another man from a different tribe, the Gwain, while he pursued an antelope he had shot. The Gwain man was also pursuing the same animal on the grounds that he too had shot it. The truth is the antelope had been hit by two arrows, obviously one from each. The Dagara man insisted he killed the antelope because he shot it first; the Gwain man claimed he saw it first and therefore must have shot it first. A fight ensued, in the course of which the Dagara tribesman killed his opponent. He then carried his game home and shared it with his family and neighbors.

It wasn't long before a strange plague hit the village. Every shaman who consulted on the issue discovered that a deep wrong had been done to a stranger in the neighboring tribe. They found out who did it, but the young man was already dead, along with some members of his family. The survivors told the story as they heard it from the young man before he died. A delegation was sent out to meet the other tribe. They confessed to the killing and paid retribution in the form of crops. In addition, the two tribes became joking partners forever. This means that every time a Dagara meets a Gwain, they must joke with each other as good old friends.

Elders refer to such righting of wrongs as "keeping the house clean for others." Thus harmony is won through cleansing and through maintaining vigilance. This allows future generations to inherit purity instead of having to repair the damage that irresponsible grandparents or great-grandparents have neglected to fix. Love of the community for the ancestors and the elders is based on and motivated by this desire for communal purity. The elders mediate in the business of continually correcting individual human lives. When an individual is called into a sacred space to right a wrong, the presence of an elder becomes the support.

Usually the correction takes the form of verbally admitting and recognizing the wrongdoing. Take, for example, a woman who promised the ancestors a gift if she was given children. Eventually she becomes the mother of four. All of them grow up in good health. But over the years, the woman has forgotten her promise. Then suddenly one of the children falls deeply ill. Every herbal medicine tried on her is not working. At last the woman has the insight to consult a shaman. There she learns she had made a promise, which she then forgot about. She goes to the ancestors' shrine and pleads for mercy: "I once came to you, O Great Ones, with a request that you bless me with fertility. At the time I was so desperate to be a mother that I was ready to trade everything I had to be one. You helped me, but my memory was short. The blessing of motherhood effaced the memory of my promise. And all these years have gone by watching me take for granted that I am a mother. And now my child is dying. You say it is because I did not fulfill my side of the bargain. I beseech you to forgive my inadvertence."

This woman's verbal admission of her wrongdoing is similar to the act of confessing sins in Christianity. Among the Dagara, this act of contrition is custom-made to suit the nature of the fault. The wrongdoer might punctuate his or her confession with metaphorical statements such as, "I bumped my leg while walking," or "My head was upside down," or "I took the wrong road." This is then followed by a statement of allegiance, in which the wrongdoer reiterates his or her close connection with the ancestors, without whom family, home, or community is impossible. Then follows the appeal to the ancestors, where the wrongdoer promises never to commit such acts again and pleads with the ancestors to forgive. The purpose of the appeal is to make the ancestors realize that they too need the wrongdoer in the interest of maintaining the community. Finally the wrongdoer presents a sacrifice or give-away to the head of the family, who presents it to the elder, who then gives it to the ancestors.

This complicated protocol is aimed at cleansing the destructive power of wrongdoing and preventing worse things from happening. The plea that the wrongdoer won't ever do anything wrong again is obviously a rhetorical statement. More often than not the people who steal from other farms would do it again. But the human potential for recidivism is not seen as cause for ostracism as long as corrective action is taken. There is some sense in which village people look at the human being as a vulnerable spirit prone to repeated falling. The important thing is not the fall, but the ability to get up boldly upon realizing that one has fallen.

We must realize here that the key thing is the give-away, not the verbal apology. Pleading guilty and saying one is sorry do not clear the air, among the Dagara. Ancestors do not accept simple words, because words are not strong enough to clear negative energy. Also, it appears that ancestors are quite aware of the extreme fallibility of humans, and their refusal to accept words as a conclusion to human problems indicates their knowledge that the words are not likely to be true. The sacrifice carries with it the power to alleviate the bad energy created by the wrongdoing because in it an animal life is offered. In traditional belief, the shedding of animal blood releases an energy for Spirit, which then takes it as a tool to wipe out the wrong and restore harmony. It is as if death, when ritualized in a clear context, contributes to life.

ELDERS, RITUALS, AND SHRINES

In addition to tending to delicate emotional situations, elders lead communal and private rituals and preside over interaction with the sacred. Because they are close to the Other World, and because they function as anchors for the village and the community, they have no difficulty overseeing the gateways to the Other World and to the ancestors. This means that the elder aims at becoming an ancestor. It is his or her next status. So there is some sense in which we can say that the elder is an ancestor in training.

The greatest responsibility of the elder is leading rituals. Among these rituals are those of birth and death. Elders welcome the newborn and say farewell to the deceased. Elders are guides for the newborn. They are the mirror through which the child can see his or her life on the human plane. Grandparents are essential to the healthy growth of our children. The fact that parents played a necessary biological role in the coming of their child does not mean that their role as primary caretakers is guaranteed to continue. In the village, more often than not this is where it ends and where the grandparents' effectiveness begins.

As mentioned earlier, the grandparent and the grandchild share something essential: their proximity to the ancestral world. The grandchild has just arrived from there, and the grandparent is heading in that direction.

Obviously they have to communicate. Because they have this in common, it becomes the focus of their relationship. The love of the grandparent for the grandchild is motivated by the fresh ancestral scent of the grandchild—something that the grandparent dreams about constantly. Similarly, the face of the grandparent is very familiar to the grandchild because it confirms to the grandchild that the world left behind is right here. This is why, among the Dagara, grandparents and grandchildren prefer to call each other brother and sister, indicating that they are almost of the same age group. In the West, where grandparents are often not present, this great resource might not be available. But perhaps the Dagara way can provide an inspiration to grandparents who would like to be more connected to their grandchildren. Perhaps also it can encourage parents of young children to include people at the far end of life in their children's lives.

Elders are also keepers of shrines. A shrine is like the ancestral Camp David, an earthly rural retreat for the ancestors. Its caretaker must in most cases be an elder or designated by an elder. It is assumed that, at any given time, an ancestor is "vacationing" at the shrine. Consequently, all amenities must be available. This includes food, aromatic herbs, and fresh drinks. The fresh items are necessary to ensure the presence of the Other World. A shrine is where one goes to enter into communication with the Other World. It is the place of beauty and mystery, and also the place of memory because shrines have the power to remind us that in human life we are at the threshold of another world. A shrine is the same as an altar. In the home, shrines always carry fresh offerings; outdoor shrines in Africa are more rugged because of the constant visits by the animals of the wild. Every house must have a shrine. It is the center of the family's identity. At these shrines, the family maintains its ongoing relationship with the ancestors. This is where gifts are offered and where prayers are formulated.

ELDERS IN THE WEST

Given the differences between indigenous and modern life, how do we recognize an elder in the West? How does one become an elder? How old are elders here?

In the culture of the West now, it is easier for someone to become an elder to their grandchildren than to anyone else because a grandchild spontaneously listens to and respects a grandparent. But I would also venture to say that there is something of an elder in any person whose words are listened to and who commands respect and attention. One should not confuse such a person with an employer who forces respect simply because a paycheck is at risk. At a number of conferences and public events, I have had the chance to witness true Western elders. They might appear in the form of an old woman whose remarks are devoutly listened to in public or an old man who commands natural respect because of his life experiences.

I vividly remember the powerful impression of an elderly woman I met in Louisiana who headed a government project. Her look and demeanor reminded me of female elders in my tribe. She carried her life experience well and spoke with poise, beauty, and wisdom. She had nothing to prove, hence her voice was never raised, but people listened. And then there was another man whose lifetime struggle with society, including several decades in and out of the prison system, made him an elder. His gravelly voice almost reminded me of a voice from the Other World. There was in it the qualities of an elder that command attention and respect.

Elders also appear as people who have profoundly changed the lives of others through their teaching or writing. In the best scenario, these teachers are able to help those who search for guidance and leadership in their lives. In the worst scenario, having become an author, they are changed into a lasting spiritual authority as well as a consumer product. In Socrates and Shakespeare, Hegel and Kierkegaard, and countless other Western

deep thinkers, we see evidence of the form in which elderhood is cultivated and practiced in the absence of a villagelike community. The Western elder is perhaps more visible as a wise thinker and holder or container
of groundbreaking initiatives in human consciousness. Hence poets,
philosophers, teachers, artists, and even social activists are either practic-
ing to become elders or have become elders altogether. Their legacy continues to affect people even as they have become, I would say, ancestors.

There is an elder in the making in everyone, but it is most visible in
those who have the receptivity to listen to the stories of others. The ability to listen, and the willingness to support others in difficult situations,
are the heart and the soul of elderhood. Young people have many difficulties to report. Anyone who would want to become an elder should lend
them a listening ear. In the life of the elder-to-be, there is very little good
news. Everyone who solicits the services of an elder-to-be is looking for a
container to unload some problems. Consequently, one can't become an
elder who would prefer to hear only the better side of life.

Similarly, anyone who attends to the sorrows of another person and
does not feel overwhelmed or frightened is a person who nurses an elder
within. To move toward the Other World, to reach the kind of durability,
stability, and anchoring strength associated with an elder, one must be
able to face the worst storms of the weather of life. This is an initiation
that cures the consciousness of its addiction to immediate rewards and allows for a slow pace to reveal life's hidden pearls. Such a person grows
into a man or a woman of resource, an elder.

Above all, to be an elder is to be able to come down to the level of the
person you listen to, not with a mind to tell that person what to do and
what not to do, but to share similar experiences you have had in the course
of your own life. People who have reached a place where they are able to
recognize that everyone has similar troubles have begun to heal. The elder does not turn the tragedy of another into a horror story, but instead
sees in the story of the other his or her connection with it.

Fame is not necessarily synonymous with being an elder. Fame often
means becoming a commodity. The person behind the fame may just be a

child starving for love and attention. But people searching for guidance tend to make famous people elders, or role models, because they have achieved something that can be seen. Because of the fluidity of information in the West, people are made mentors or elders without physical contact. The mentor and the elder are both in high demand. Both can be found in the same person, but not always. A mentor may need an elder, but an elder does not need a mentor. In this culture, where the quest for both the elder and the mentor is almost epidemic, it is not surprising that a person able to mentor is made prematurely into an elder.

I still remember the great shift in attitude toward me when I published my first book. People who, prior to that, would question, act suspiciously, or even reject what I said began suddenly to accept almost indiscriminately anything from me. One problem with the authority that authorship confers is that it has something irreversible about it. This authority can suddenly turn a person into a mentor or an elder. It is as if in the Western context these roles arise as a result of an event in the person's life that brings that person to a certain level of visibility.

ELDERS AND THE SACRED

If people in the West embraced the idea that the elder is at the edge, between two worlds, and is therefore a window to the Other World as well as a mirror of it, certain of the West's social problems would be solved. One of them is the rejection of aging and the elders, which puts the culture at risk. The other is the West's relationship to the sacred.

There is no doubt that in Western culture, the fear of aging has become quite acute. People certainly have many reasons to think that old age is not something to look forward to. But in light of what has been said about elders in an indigenous African context, one could explain Western fear of old age as linked to the sense of uselessness. If in Western society people would find ways in their old age of spending their abundant time with their grandchildren, perhaps this would raise the appreciation of old age and pave the road for a more sacred approach to being old. For if to get old is to get close to the ancestors, then old means that which is closest to the sacred.

If a culture rejects the sacred, it rejects elders. If it rejects elders, it rejects the welfare of its youth. You can't have the one without the other. It is understood in the village that youth and the elders are the ones in society who see clearly what is happening. The young are at an age where the hidden is obvious to their eyes. They want to point it out because they do not know how to pretend it is not there.

To be young or old in the modern world is to be at risk. People who wish to embrace their elderhood must first listen to the pain around them. They must notice in the young and the adult the parts that are craving visibility. We must learn how to sit quietly with our youth and to listen quietly to what they have to say. This is the job of elders. This calm, almost meditative approach to youth can also be a model for self-calming to other people who are too troubled to be quiet. Calmness is the beginning of the ability to hold the space, the beginning of an elder's contribution to the community.

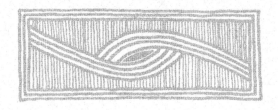

PART THREE

UNDERSTANDING

RITUAL

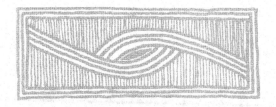

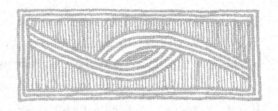

7.

The Elements
of Ritual

I would rediscover the secret of great
communications and great combustions. I would
say storm. I would say river. I would say tornado.
I would say leaf. I would say tree. I would be
drenched by all rain, moistened by all dews. I
would roll like frenetic blood on the slow current
of the eye of words turned into mad horses into
fresh children into clots into vestiges of temples
into precious stones remote enough to discourage
miners. Whoever would not understand me would
not understand any better the roaring of a tiger.
—AIMÉ CÉSAIRE, *Notebook of a Return to the*
Native Land, translated by Clayton Eshleman
and Annette Smith

Ritual is the most ancient way of binding a
community together in a close relationship
with Spirit. It is a way of communicating
with forms of consciousness and beings

from countless worlds. It has been one of the most practical and efficient ways to stimulate the safe healing required by both the individual and the community. Ritual has always been the way of life of the spiritual person because it is a tool to maintain the delicate balance between body and soul. In a tribal community, healing of the village happens in ritual.

WHAT IS RITUAL?

Every time a gathering of people, under the protection of Spirit, triggers a body of emotional energy aimed at bringing them very tightly together, a ritual of one type or another is in effect. In this kind of gathering people primarily use nonverbal means of interacting with one another, thereby stimulating the life of the psyche. What happened in the United States when President Kennedy was assassinated can be likened to a ritual. Suddenly and spontaneously, the country came together, bound by an emotional energy. In the indigenous context, death triggers the same ritual response. When someone dies, everything stops and the village comes together for the funeral.

There are two parts to ritual. One part is planned: people prepare the space for the ritual and think through the general choreography of the process. The other part of ritual cannot be planned because it is the part that Spirit is in charge of. The unplanned part of ritual is a spontaneous, almost unpredictable interaction with an energy source. It is a response to a call from a nonhuman source to commune with a larger horizon. It is like a journey. Before you get started, you own the journey. After you start, the journey owns you.

Certain events move us irresistibly toward ritualized behaviors, for example the loss of a loved one, a major accident, the witnessing of a violent death, or a natural disaster. When such an event happens, no observer can predict people's actions or logically explain what goes on, because the people affected by the event act without conscious control. Any emotional frenzy, to the extent that it is orchestrated by Spirit, has something ritualistic about it. Ritual can look like an opportunity for loss of control, the place where you surrender your control to Spirit—to whatever force is present—because you trust the leadership of that force. Even highly controlled people, from time to time, want to cut loose. Ritual offers this opportunity, for in ritual you may be able to plan what will happen, but you cannot plan the outcome. This is because people will respond in spontaneous ways to the call of Spirit, and where exactly the journey will take the group, no one can say.

It is important to recognize what ritual is not. It is not repetitive or compulsive behavior, like having coffee or a cigarette in the morning. Nor is it an everyday formality, like greeting another person with a handshake, hug, or kiss. In day-to-day life, when you go to a public place of business, you are expected to stand in line if you find that others have preceded you to the same place. Ritual is just the opposite. It is gathering with others in order to feel Spirit's call, to express spontaneously and publicly whatever emotion needs to be expressed, to create, in concert with others, an unrehearsed and deeply moving response to Spirit, and to feel the presence of the community, including the ancestors, throughout the experience.

People's psyches are very drawn to ritual because it's a place of high ecstasy. What happens in ritual is not unlike what happens to people who ingest drugs. Ritual is a place of safe ecstasy, but with no undesirable side effects. This is one of the reasons why indigenous people love ritual. They spend the majority of their time planning for ritual, doing it, and recovering from it.

It is important also to distinguish between ritual and ceremony. I remember the first time I was invited to a wedding in the West. I thought it would be an opportunity to see a true ritual, since two people were going to be melted into wedlock for life. I was thinking about the deeply ritualistic event that a wedding implies in my own culture. There, a whole family escorts a bride to the groom after making an offer at the altar of the ancestors. At the groom's house the ritual welcoming begins with another gathering of the elders at the shrine of the groom's ancestors. The invocation prayer is aimed at protection, good health, children, and harmony.

They offer sacrifices of chickens, pour water for peace and continued reconciliation, then distribute ash for protection against bad spirits. After
this, the bride's village must sing songs of praise to the bride and demand
that the groom's village and family members prove their worthiness. For
long hours a chanted dialogue occurs between villages and families,
where the bride's people investigate in songs the economic, social, and
political worth of the groom's people. The bride's people will not enter
the groom's house for the first refreshment of the day until satisfied that
the groom's people check out well on every item. Of course they know all
this in advance, but, as when a priest or minister asks a bride and a groom
if they want to take each other as partners, knowing what the answer will
be, the responses need to be made public.

When I was invited to an American wedding I was still carrying my
culturally shaped ideas about the kind of ritual that the wedding would
be. That is why I was disappointed. First, I admired the beautiful clothing
that nearly everybody wore. The bride looked angelic in her white dress.
The groom was a true gentleman, beautiful in his black tuxedo. But the
beauty of the participants was not enough to constitute a moving ritual.
To me, the crowd's attitude was most strange. The passivity of those present made me wonder if anyone cared about the bride and the groom. People seemed more responsive to appearances, drinks, and partying than to
the sacred commitment of the two getting married. The exchange of
vows had little sincerity, except in the case of the bride, who seemed to
carry some emotion in her answer, "I do." But the vows seemed to emphasize the heavy burdens placed upon the couple. Each was asked if they
promised to love the other whether sick or healthy, miserable or happy,
wealthy or poor. They both said "Yes." The crowd said nothing.

My first reaction was, "This is not possible. Two people can't do this
alone." I was instinctively responding to the fact that in my culture, the
families exchange the wedding vows on behalf of the couple. The essence
of this collective vow is the recognition that the ancestors are witnesses to
the couple's commitment to serve and care for each other. These same an-

cestors will counsel the two families in times of stress as much as in times of joy.

From an indigenous point of view, ceremonies are events that are reproducible, predictable, and controllable, while rituals call for spontaneous feeling and trust in the outcome. The annual Rose Parade in Pasadena on New Year's Day has no space for the spontaneity and disorder that accompany the emotional surrender of ritual. The Memorial Day service in Arlington National Cemetery will not authorize spontaneity. Anyone who burst into tears and audible cries, for example, would probably be considered a disruption. These events are ceremonies, not rituals.

Ritual, by contrast, is a time of unplanned, unforeseeable, yet orderly disorder. Whereas in ceremony there is a potential for boredom because the participants pretty much know what's going to happen, in ritual the soul and the human spirit get permission to express themselves.

What to Westerners are rituals appear to indigenous people as instead ceremonies. Among the most visible expressions are the varieties of church practices, from Mass to processional celebrations. When I was a teenager living in a Catholic seminary, I especially used to appreciate candlelight ceremonies on Easter night. The otherworldliness of the service was extremely attractive to me. On Ash Wednesday, I liked the touch of ash on my forehead, although I blocked out the words "You are ash and shall return to ash." The problem with these ceremonies is that over time they begin to lose their attraction, since they happen in the same way year after year. They do not have the essential ingredient, spontaneity, which to indigenous people speaks of the presence of Spirit. Of course, the same words said in the same way over time do help many people in the West feel connected to Spirit because the very repetition reminds people of the thousands who have gone before who said the same words and so must have gone through a similar experience. But the presence of Spirit is marked in African villages in just the opposite way—by releasing emotion spontaneously rather than by providing a container for emotion through familiar words.

When most Westerners think of ritual, they are more likely to connect it with words such as *empty, old-fashioned, irrelevant,* and *boring* than with words such as *transforming, essential, challenging,* or *healing.* Ritual continues to engage the passion and commitment of indigenous people because it stimulates their creativity and their emotions. Most of all, they continue to do ritual because afterward they feel changed. Doing ritual heals people, reconnecting them to the ancestors and to their own deepest purpose. Because ritual is so deeply connected to our human nature, anytime it is missing there will be a lack of transformation and healing. If a culture does not draw from ritual, its members will do something else to fill the gap because they have to heal. In the absence of ritual, Westerners turn instead to therapists, self-help groups, or, at a more destructive end of the spectrum, to alcohol and drugs.

Ritual is a dance with Spirit, the soul's way of interacting with the Other World, the human psyche's opportunity to develop relationship with the symbols of this world and the spirits of the other.

SYMBOLS: THE DOORWAY TO RITUAL

Symbols are the doorway to ritual. Just as our bodies can't survive without nourishment, our psyches cannot sustain themselves without symbolism. For example, when people look at the Vietnam War Memorial in Washington, D.C., they are in awe, deeply moved. This is the expression of their psyche's relationship with the symbol that is embodied there. You can't afford to be superficial or casual in the face of this symbol. It's as if all the dead of the Vietnam War were behind that monument, and the psyche sees them, feels them, and communicates with them, as they see, feel, and communicate with us. A similar function is played by a national flag. In itself it is just a piece of painted cloth, but because this cloth represents a nation, the cloth is honored by some, who salute it, and effaced by others, who want the nation to change. From this we may recognize that a key element of ritual is symbolism.

In just about any of the seven thousand villages that make up the country of Burkina Faso, the most noticeable cultural element is the symbol. From the way human dwellings are built to the smallest visual representation, forms that represent something greater in another world are very important. To enter many villages and towns, one must go through an archlike vault, making a person feel that they are crossing over from one realm to another. As I travel from village to village in Dagara territory, what catches my attention more than anything else are the crosslike monuments at the front door of many dwellings. It is as if something other than my eyes notices these things. These monuments are dedicated to the ancestors. They are an expression of the inseparable connection with the dead and with Spirit. Villages where Christianity has taken hold have fewer of these monuments. The houses that carry them are not yet converted.

A few years ago I was traveling with a cousin to a remote village in a hilly area near the border with Ghana. As we approached the small settlement, my cousin stopped suddenly. "Stop breathing," he said breathlessly. I was going to ask why, but realized he was not ready to answer. His body was soaking wet with perspiration, and he was shivering, while looking everywhere as if he expected something to burst out of nowhere. His eyes rolled from one side to the other, and then circled around their orbit deliberately trying to lock on to something. I waited.

It was not long before he walked straight to a little bush, moved a few leafy branches away, and unveiled a form that at first did not make sense to me. It was clearly humanly made and in an unusual place. People do not build things like this in the bush unless there is a very serious reason. It was a monument to a being from the Other World. Judging by the freshness of chicken feathers and blood clots around the area, people had left the place not long before my cousin unveiled it. He bent down in a long bow to the sacred representation. I did the same. He said some words that I did not hear very well, but that I understood as an explanation of our purpose in visiting the village. Then he took out some cowrie shells and dropped them there before we proceeded into the village.

It took me a while before I began to understand what had happened.

My cousin's psyche had picked up the presence of a sacred symbol with which he had a connection. Indeed, this monument was the representation of a particular being from a different world, a *kontomblé*, with whom he had a relationship. Anytime, anywhere he came near this symbol, his psyche noticed it at once, and it was his duty to pay tribute. I remembered that, at the time, I was disturbed mostly because my cousin was disturbed, not because my own psyche had perceived anything.

Some time later my cousin and I were talking about these beings from another world. Remembering that I had been blind to their presence, I asked how his psyche had been able to see them and mine had not. He said: "Yours did too, you just did not pay attention." I didn't think he understood that I, as a sincere seeker of Spirit, would not have overlooked such presences. So I objected. He laughed and insisted that this is what had happened. I began to think, Could it be that the human psyche has eyes that see things independently of the physical eyes? How is it that inner sight and outer awareness do not always coincide? I could recall being in places where I felt unexplainable chills, but I thought it was just a physiological reaction.

The example of my cousin shows that the human psyche "reads" symbols; it is symbol literate or symbol sensitive. That is, the psyche recognizes symbols wherever they are and reacts to them at all times. We may refer to symbols and our reactions to them in more comfortable terms such as instinct or intuition, but beneath this is the recognition that a separate entity in us experiences reality in ways different from the way the conscious self perceives the world.

The psyche that lacks this grounding is easily depressed. Finding meaning in life requires focusing the psyche toward a reality that extends beyond the everyday world, and the human psyche requires symbols to maintain that focus. Symbols refer us to the Other World; they make us aware of that world, the world from which we draw our deepest connection and identity. Symbols are, as it were, messages pointing to a different and higher dimension, or consciousness. The part of the self that craves this reality will recognize it through symbols.

This is one of the reasons why ancient places attract visitors. Among the tourists are people whose spirits are so awake that they feel pulled to these places in order to renew their ties to the Other World. I have heard stories from people who have been to ancient sites and could not resist the overwhelming and strange feelings that washed over them, or who burst into tears, or who even experienced an unusual sense of familiarity with the space. There are rational explanations for this, but there is another type of explanation related to the soul's timeless recognition of its affinity with an area, a place, or a monument.

The symbolic and the spiritual are not far apart. In fact, in Dagara, there is no word that directly translates as *symbol*. There is no word for symbol other than the word *Spirit*, because there is an assumed indivisible connection between Spirit and symbol. Beings that live in other dimensions are so intimately linked to us that they are referred to by name. They are not considered mere metaphors or abstract representations of intangible concepts. These beings simply live in a different time/space continuum and perceive us as much as we perceive them. They refer to our world as the Other World and see us as spirits, which is why they are interested in us. They are living, as it were, on the other side of the page of our reality. The Western view of different planes of existence may be helpful in understanding what I am referring to here. Another bridging image is the notion of fields of energy in quantum physics. In quantum physics, the understanding of matter as transferable to energy suggests a flexible attitude toward the nature and limits of the visible and material world.

For the Dagara and other indigenous people, it is inconceivable that the human mind could capture something that does not already exist somewhere. The human capacity to imagine is an example of our connection with remote fields of energy. If human consciousness is able to capture, and thereby understand, these realities, then imagination and visionary consciousness are linking us to other types of realities, directly or otherwise. If modern consciousness is, for the time being, unable to interact with other intelligences in the time-space continuum, the modern psyche nevertheless maintains a great attraction toward and relationship with other dimensions and types of consciousness.

How is this visionary ability connected to ritual? In the indigenous mind, one reason people do ritual is that they do not want to repeat history, dealing constantly with unfinished business from the past. The appeal to the ancestors through ritual is based on an understanding that catastrophe happens when you fail to seek their guidance. So in some ways, doing ritual is like preventing the self from falling into destructive patterns. The symbolic spiritual realm speaks to the psyche the same way that a travel guidebook speaks to the conscious self—it confirms our location. Human beings need these reminders on the journey of life; they are the billboards of the psyche.

TYPES OF RITUAL

Two types of rituals are commonly practiced among the Dagara. The first one is called *radical ritual* because it involves major repair of the broken or damaged human psyche or spirit. In such a ritual, the physical body is pushed to the extreme in order to create a situation of tension favorable for the removal of unwanted energetic debris and the restoration of a much more acceptable self. The second one is called *maintenance ritual*. It is a nonstressful yet regular practice of acknowledging an existing connection with the Other World, the world of Spirit. This is based on the assumption that normal life produces some wear and tear to the spiritual self and, by extension, to the physical self.

The most prominent kind of ritual is the radical ritual, because it involves community. Radical ritual is a dramatic interaction with Spirit for the purpose of removing from the psyche something that has been seriously troublesome to a person in the village. For example, a person who is torn by a physical or a psychological problem, who suffers from abandonment, low self-esteem or paranoia, or who is a victim of severe abuse, will require one, if not several, radical rituals. The ritual will push out the energy that is keeping him or her trapped and will open a new space to fill with the appropriate energy. This kind of ritual cannot be done by one person. It must be done by the community for the person. Dagara funeral rituals are radical rituals, primarily because they aim at unloading the huge emotional flood stored in people's souls as a result of the sudden parting of a loved one. The death of a loved one leaves an energy thread that binds the living with an emotional debt. It is as if the thread that ties people together becomes a source of pain when someone dies. In order to heal from it and to free both parties, one must let go of the thread. Thus it is difficult to release the dead without a major ritual outburst.

Once you have rid yourself of such a paralyzing emotional energy and, with the help of the community, have replaced it with a more balanced feeling, you need a maintenance ritual. It's like a three-month, three-thousand-mile oil change. No major repairs to do, just maintenance. A maintenance ritual is focused on making sure that all the nuts and bolts of one's spirit are still in place, holding together the physical self. In it, all that is required is a full-hearted prayer to the spirit guides thanking them for their presence and requesting that they stay nearby in order to lead in the day ahead. You state what is ahead, the tasks you are facing, and request the ongoing assistance of the ancestors or any spirit ally you know.

A person who is in charge of other people's needs, a counselor for example, will need some kind of daily ritual to restore their psyche after long hours of devotion to the good of others. Otherwise, over time the psyche will develop major "mechanical" problems. The maintenance ritual is intended to keep one in a normal running condition. It is self-care at the level of the spirit.

THE RITUAL PROCESS

There are usually four components to a ritual:

1. Preparing the Ritual Space. A ritual space is a place loaded with symbolism, capable of keeping the psyche focused away from the turbu-

lence of everyday life. It must be a place outside of the ordinary, a place that looks and feels like an oasis in the middle of the desert. The requirements for a ritual space include an overwhelming dose of beauty and mystery. The symbolic is usually mysterious to the ordinary mind, but it is perfectly understandable to the psyche. In preparing the ritual space, keep in mind that there must be a way to tell where the space begins and where it ends because a ritual space is sacred. The gateway into the sacred space should be obvious. These features help the psyche to make the transition between this world and the one afforded by the sacred.

Since the exact ingredients needed to make the ritual successful cannot be known before the ritual occurs, it is useful to include representations of all the elements (water, fire, earth, nature, and mineral) in the symbolic items that decorate the space. Including all the elements reminds everyone that any or all of the essences of these elements may be needed to accomplish the purpose of the ritual. (The elements are discussed in more detail in chapters 9 through 13.) The inclusion of a small personal object from each individual involved in the ritual serves to remind each person of his or her connection to the sacred space that has been created.

2. The Invocation. The invocation is a form of prayer that formally invites Spirit, or any kind of personal deity, to join or participate in what is about to happen. For ritual to be a ritual, Spirit, the divine, or any allied force from a world different from ours must be present to guide and move the ritual to the right destination. Spirits come when they are invited, and they come with a lot of friends, distant relatives and their friends.

For a culture that keeps Spirit outside of its day-to-day operation, any invitation of Spirit produces a rush from the Other World. So the invocation must be very specific as to who is wanted and who is not, and the purpose of the invitation needs to be made explicit. For instance, rather than simply inviting the spirit of Mother Earth to come and be present, it would be more useful to ask, "Spirit of Mother Earth, come and hold our feet to the ground while we try and deal with the difficult problems we face today, and provide for us from your abundance as we enter a period of some great upheaval and change." Each individual needs a chance to invite those spirits important to them and to state their intent for the ritual that is about to occur. By stating the purpose of the ritual in the invocation, and by making it clear that you are not inviting these spirits for something vain, you determine who will come and who will not. I am implying here that there are good and bad spirits, spirits that are useful and spirits that are not useful to us. Vagueness is interpreted by bad spirits as an invitation to participate in our activities. But narrowing down our intent eliminates these risks and enhances the chance that the spirits that come will be actively involved with the task we have laid out.

In the invocation we acknowledge the fact that we are almost helpless in the face of the illnesses and problems that cripple us. In fact, the invocation is our opportunity to show how humble we are, or are willing to be, in the interest of allowing change to happen. There must be a total willingness to put aside preconceived ideas about what the outcome of the ritual should be, with no restrictions placed beforehand on the range of possible outcomes. This allows the open mind necessary to hear and see whatever is revealed in the course of the ritual, with the willingness to do whatever it takes to bring about healing.

For example, we can say at the beginning of a ritual involving fire, "O ancestors, we humbly ask that you join us today as we face this uncertain task of burning up the things that keep us from experiencing true communion with you. Please make use of our arms that they may perform the right gestures. Take over our eyes that they may look where you order them to look, and see what needs to be seen. Enter into our feet that they may walk at the right pace on the journey to healing. Take over our bodies that they may bow to the healing you're bringing to us."

The sincere invocation of Spirit and the subsequent surrender of the ritual process to Spirit suggests that whatever happens will be determined by Spirit. This is because we understand that the purpose of the ritual cannot be achieved by us; we do not have the skills or the knowledge to do that. Ritual is an activity for change. In order for the change to be genuine and lasting, there must be a Spirit intervention. The invocation relieves the person who is conducting the ritual from the painful task of having to decide what comes next in the ritual. We recognize this process in Western culture when we say, "Wherever the spirit leads." This requires a lot of trust, and the willingness to let go of control. Healing happens when we surrender our control to Spirit, who is the real healer.

3. Healing. The healing section of the ritual process is key to the success of the ritual itself. If nothing happens here, then a ritual did not happen. Healing does not come packaged the way we would like. For anything to happen at all we must open up, and be on the watch, for the pull of Spirit. Too much inhibition or self-criticism or analysis scrambles the call from Spirit to get involved. We are easily distracted by passing thoughts and sensations; we miss the subtle pull to actions, that is, the appropriate but instinctual move that heals. We must test our listening ability to see if it can include the low-frequency waves of other planes. What I mean is that healing includes hearing the sound that can move us to surrender to healing. This assumes that music plays a significant part in healing because it allows our spirits to be transported to where we need to be for the right thing to occur. When healing takes place, unforeseen things occur. The person looking for healing may suddenly experience things in such a way that his or her actions are almost uncontrollable. This is why, more often than not, the healing part of the ritual contains a lot of emotion.

Emotion is certainly perceivable when Spirit is present. In some cases it moves people to emit sounds and move their bodies in ways that are unusual and unfamiliar. It may in the extreme make some people act as if they are possessed, and this can frighten others who may not understand what is going on. The problem is that we need to grasp the logic of emotion fully in order not to be frightened by it. A person who breaks down in the middle of a ritual has become some sort of vessel through which spirit is doing the work we requested. Therefore the emotion that one feels in a ritual space is the healing energy stirred up by Spirit. Allowing one's emotion to expand means accepting a much-needed healing. The more clearly people's emotions are expressed, the more clearly they are involved with the healing spirits.

More often than not, when the healing section is reached, people's resistance drops, and they move from self-consciousness to self-awareness. The self-conscious mind often stiffens in the territory of healing because this is an uncharted place. In contrast, the self-aware has given up its stiffness. When you're self-conscious, your approach to reality is colored by a rather high dose of criticism. When you are self-aware, you start doing things that are not logically explicable, things the mind can't justify, and that the self-conscious mind would love to criticize. This is why in the healing section, in order to allow the purpose to be accomplished, it is important for participants to be willing to reorient the ritual if necessary, following its path of intensity rather than letting it go in a wrong direction.

I remember a ritual that was allowed to wander from its healing course. This ritual was aimed at cleansing the self, but it turned into some strange get-together to share personal wounds. The group was supposed to gather at a place that had been cleaned up for that purpose. While singing and dancing, each person was invited, as he or she felt ready, to walk to a place where they were helped by a team of helpers to apply earth on the part of their bodies that needed cleansing. After this, they were guided to another place, where they were dipped into water, and then they were escorted back to the original place. The invocation was beautiful. It stressed our vulnerability to contagion and pleaded for the Great Spirits to assist in the release of any impurity we may carry. Then came the healing part. We chanted in cadence with the beat of a drum. People began walking through the process. After a while, I noticed that the journey from the earth to the water was not happening. I went and found out that the helpers at the earth place were not doing their job. Everyone that came in to seek their help was enrolled into something like a therapy session. The crowd waiting to apply earth to their bodies was growing bigger and bigger. I had to interrupt and tell them what needed to be done to provide fluidity. The interruption provided an opportunity for the ritual to intensify, once people began to complete their journey from the earth place to the water place and then back to the starting point.

Because of our tendency to assert control, we need to be aware that our controlling self may try to kick in during ritual. One signal that this has happened is the feeling that the ritual has become more like theater, with an embarrassing superficiality. In a play, people go into scripted rage and weep synchronized tears. The display of emotion is recognized as unreal but is welcomed nonetheless because its purpose is simply to entertain. In ritual, the actor can creep in quite easily too. It is the duty of the ritual leader to rid the process from any such pretense, even at the risk of becoming the target of inflamed criticism. This is why in the village elders are so important, for they can stop a ritual that is not healing, while anyone else who tries to do so is likely to be attacked.

This is not to say that acting is always bad in ritual. The key is genuineness of purpose; every action needs to be focused toward the pure intention of seeking healing. In order for an individual to experience change, the whole group involved in the ritual must contribute focused and coordinated attention and energy to the individual. This is why most of the time people sing together, dance together, and drum together.

There are no prescriptions for the content of the healing section of the ritual. The problem for which healing is sought and the healing that is needed are usually defined in terms of one of the five elements. Generally the clan of people associated with the element whose energy is needed determine the actual structure of the ritual, asking for and relying on the help of Spirit to guide the planning. Often the entire group that will participate in the ritual assists in the planning, with the act of planning itself becoming a small ritual. There is usually an elder present who has responsibility for overseeing the ritual, assuring that all the necessary elements are present, that the important details have been attended to. It is rarely the case that a single person plans the entire ritual, like a teacher with a lesson plan coming to a classroom full of students. The planning itself can be as exciting and healing as the ritual itself. In it you can see how various imaginations come together to focus on the issue that the ritual is intended to address. Differences arise, and people learn how not to be too attached to what they think should be the way the ritual should go.

4. The Closing. A ritual that begins well must be closed, and closed well. The closing is an expression of gratitude for what the presence of Spirit has allowed to happen. Just as the invocation consists mainly in asking Spirit to be actively present, the closing is an opportunity to acknowledge the good that has been brought forth through the agency of Spirit. It is important to be as detailed as possible in this section. You can't simply say thank you; it is very important to itemize the things that you are thankful for. This means that the ritual leader must watch the changes unfolding in everyone. These changes are not of the same nature in each person or in every ritual. Some are collective changes, others—most of them—are individual. As many as possible of the changes must be named and the Spirit thanked for them. At the conclusion of this outpouring of gratitude, the spirits must be released but not ordered to leave. A release is a simple announcement that their purpose-oriented involvement has ended. So in this case, Spirit is told to go if Spirit wants to, or to stay around if it wishes to continue inspiring us to more beauty.

RITUAL EXPERIENCES

At a retreat in California focused on ritual, a small group of thirty-five people, maybe forty, came together in planning and conducting a water ritual. We designated it a radical ritual, because it involved a whole community and because we were seeking deep healing. We called it a water ritual because its purpose was to help those with unreconciled matters in their life, reconciliation being the gift or attribute of water.

At the retreat site, we found a little stream. The water wasn't very deep, but it was quite clean. Twenty feet from the stream we cleared a space that we designated as the village. It was the place where everyone would gather during the ritual. The village was carefully marked off and was decorated to look beautiful. At the center of it we laid a fire ring ready to ignite. It was to symbolize the collective focus. The village was facing the stream where the radical ritual was to take place. As you walked toward the stream from the village you had to pass through a gateway. It was built with natural elements, including ferns and flowers, and was intended to symbolize a gateway between the village and the healing place of the stream. Close to the stream was another gateway, smaller in size but just as impressive and beautiful.

The water was decorated to look, when night came, like a place of light, and to inspire people to devotion and piety. The reflection of countless candles floated in it with the kind of gentleness that invokes trust, safety, and even love. From the village to the healing place of the stream, the path was paved with dancing light.

We divided into three groups, each with a specific function in the village. One group was in charge of the village dynamic. In addition to building the space for the village, these people were expected to keep everyone singing and moving throughout the ritual. The second group was in charge of the healing. Their headquarters was at the waterfront, even though only a few at a time actually stood there during the ritual. The third group was in charge of the overall fluidity of the ritual. They worked on the gateways and the road to the waters, planting all the candles we needed to make it look beautiful in the dark. All three groups worked hard during the day.

When night came, we proceeded to the village, chanting and drumming. The atmosphere was tense, but also comforting because people were eager to benefit from what they had invested so much energy in preparing. At the village we prayed to Spirit, asking for help in finding peace amid the rattling of the world, and of everyday life. We asked Spirit to come and help us align within. When the invocation was complete, the healers walked to the stream and waited for the first person to come. I must refrain from describing details of what happened at the waterfront out of respect for the ritual itself, and for the people who participated in it. It suffices to stress the fact that there was a huge emotional release that healed most of the people who walked the short distance to the stream and surrendered to the helpers there.

As soon as the first person returned from the stream and crossed the gateway into the village, the fire was lit. It burst into flames, as if excited by the state of the returning villager. Each returning villager was accompanied by two helpers, one posted on either side. As the fire grew, the drummer kicked in with a frenetic rhythm, and the village burst into an African song of praise to the ancestors, a Dagara song that we had all learned together earlier. For five hours we sang and drummed in support of those who went to the stream seeking help in reconciling with the plethora of things they were in conflict with in their day-to-day lives. At first the singing was rather formal. But as time progressed it became more and more emotionally intense and physically relaxed. People began to dance, some alone, others holding hands. Each person that returned to the village after being healed at the stream broke into tears as he or she was welcomed by everybody else. Some were weeping long before they were escorted back to the village. Their tears intensified upon their return. When it all ended, we were in such a high, and we thanked the Spirit with great emphasis. It was past midnight. Tired, though full of joy, we went to sleep.

The next morning people shared their experience of the ritual. A great number of them found it one of the most transforming experiences of their lives. Some were still in the emotion of their experience. They spoke in tears about how they felt. What it taught me is that ritual works wherever there is enough openness and receptivity. It works where people are willing to suspend for the moment their own disbelief and lack of clarity about the actual mechanics and logic of ritual.

Here is another idea for a group ritual: It gathers any number of people indoors. They are divided into three groups. The first group is made of people who are at the start of a challenge in their life—anything from starting a new career to facing a disturbing lawsuit or discovering that one is terminally ill. The second group includes those who are in the middle of a challenge or an ordeal. This could be a lingering bad relationship that won't heal or a painful journey. And the third group includes those who are at the tail end of an ordeal.

Each group gathers together at a central altar that all have built together for their ritual. One of them serves as facilitator. Each person takes the time to formulate his or her problem into a prayer directed at Spirit, and in which he or she is as detailed as possible. Then the facilitator leads the rest of the group into a prayer on behalf of the person. At the end of each prayer the group sings together. The song is a milestone between the previous and the next prayer. It weaves them together and becomes the tool for closing the ritual.

In families and small communities, one of the most adequate rituals for resolving issues that arise between members is referred to as an ash ritual. It is called this because in it you use ash to draw a line or to make a circle. The people with issues walk into this circle and face each other, while everyone else sits outside, also facing one another. The person who called for the ash ritual speaks his or her truth about what is hurting. The emphasis is not on blame, but on how the actions of the other have resulted in hurt and bad feeling. The other person responds, emphasizing the motive of his or her action. The people present support them by guiding them away from accusatory language, such as "You did this and I don't like your guts," and so forth. Usually a healthy imparting of one's feeling to the other results in cathartic understanding, and the whole session ends in embrace.

WHY RITUAL?

In summary, why is ritual important? As much as our body requires food for nourishment, our souls and spirits require ritual to stay whole. It is as if without the spirit being nourished in us, the body pays for the consequences. The food of the psyche is the symbol, and it is through ritual that our spirit is fed. Because human beings are spirits at our core, it is natural for us to remain mindful of our true spiritual identity.

Ritual is also necessary because there are certain problems that cannot be resolved with words alone. The pain of abuse that someone carries within, the trauma of unfulfilled dreams, and the sorrow of loss are not the kind of feelings that go away over time. Whether we deny them or not, they remain as part of the weight that keeps our bodies tensed and our spirits constricted. They fuel our drive to violence, and they eat our spirit. When they are addressed in ritual, however, we get the chance to heal them. Ritual offers the opportunity to relieve a tension from which words can no longer release us. Perhaps a great number of social issues can be resolved not by creating more institutions but by creating rituals tailored to suit them. Complex problems plague and cripple entire communities; by actively involving the members of the community in seeking solutions based in ritual, a community can achieve a deeper solution than words and rhetoric alone can provide. Breaking the spell of circular arguments through the power of ritual is an area where indigenous people can provide effective help to the West.

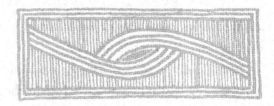

8.

Dagara Cosmology
and Ritual

Two cultures seem to intermingle in a fascinating,
ambiguous embrace only so that each can inflict
on the other a more visible denial.
—MICHEL LEIRIS, *Frêle Brut*

Cultures define themselves in terms of the
ways their people perceive the cosmos. Religions such as Christianity, Islam, Bud-
dhism, and Hinduism are born out of this
perception. The cosmology I am concerned
with in this chapter is so essential to Dagara
wisdom that little makes sense without it;
the cosmology is the foundational model
for life itself. It reveals much about indigenous people's awareness of how intimately
we are connected to creation and nature.

Dagara cosmology is the starting point of tribal ritual and is thus the sustaining principle of tribal life.

Ritual rises out of a certain understanding of the universe, how it is put together, how it functions, and where the human being fits in its evolution. The concept of evolution may be recent in the West, but to indigenous Africans it is ancient. There is a clear sense of biological change in Dagara cosmology; however, the Darwinian notion of the survival of the fittest does not appear. Instead the Dagara perceive that natural elements in their transformational progress have affected consciousness and biology in fundamental ways.

THE COSMOS AS A WHEEL

In Dagara cosmology, the image and structure of the circle, or wheel, organizes perceptions of the world (see Figure 1, p. 165). The wheel not only refers to the cyclic nature of life, but it is also a microcosm of the circular nature of the planet where we live. The indigenous tendency therefore is to perceive all of life within the context of this circular cycle, or cosmology.

When something of cosmic proportion occurs, such as an earthquake, plague, or drought, seeing it as part of a wheel or as a cosmological message determines the approach and attitude toward it. In the West, by contrast, where progress is seen as a linear journey into the future, a natural catastrophe is approached as an unfortunate obstacle. The reaction is to fix the problem by removing the obstacle and then move on. The results are regarded as damage or cost and are measured in terms of dollars and cents. The event is seen as an attack, an insurgency, that must be quickly countered, stepped over, and relegated to the past of a linear history. For example an earthquake in Los Angeles that downs bridges and homes is quickly answered by an almost instant rebuilding. It is as if people cannot tolerate the directness of Mother Earth's message to us. It must be erased

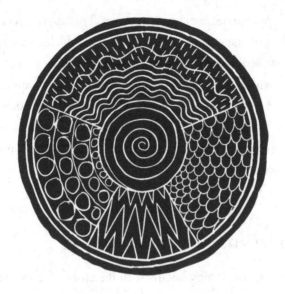

Figure 1 (©1998 Richard Martin)
The medicine wheel of the Dagara people is a symbolic representation of the
relationships between the five elements that form the cosmos. Earth is at the
center and touches all of the other elements. Water is in the North, opposite Fire,
in the South. Mineral lies in the West, and Nature is in the East. The color of Fire
is red; the color of Earth is yellow; the color of Mineral is white; the color of Water
is blue or black; and the color of Nature is green.

as quickly as possible because it comes as an interference to the forward
motion of civilization. This is a logical reaction to a linear view of life.

An indigenous African interpretation would be that the shaking of the
earth is a message to us. We may not understand it at first, which does not
mean that we should ask Mother Earth to repeat what she already said so
eloquently, but we must come down on our knees with prayers of con-
sternation and mourning, expressing the willingness to understand that
this event in the natural world and our lives are connected. Meanwhile village life is suspended until all prescribed rituals are done. Then recon-

struction, if appropriate, can begin in peace. This approach is based on an understanding of the cyclical nature of life, in which everything that exists in time and space—the earth, the moon, and other planets—is part of a continuous wheel and is connected to everything that happens. An event that is not addressed properly, that is cosmologically, is bound to happen again in a more forceful tone because it needs to be understood and adequately replied to, not silenced or ignored. This is why cosmology is key to indigenous life and spirituality.

CREATION AND THE FIVE ELEMENTS

For the Dagara, cosmology begins with the story of creation. In the beginning there was no earth as we know it. In its place was a burning planet, a ball of fire combusting at high speed. Therefore, fire is the first element of the Dagara wheel. Fire is present in everything, and everything needs fire. It was not until this moving and burning sphere encountered a huge body of water that things began to change. Water became the second element in the cosmological wheel. The shock resulting from the collision of fire and water not only slowed the combustion process, but also chased fire into the underworld, leaving the surface as a hot steamy place, fertile for the breeding of all kinds of life forms. This surface, hospitable to life, is what is known as earth, which constitutes the third elemental principle of the Dagara cosmological wheel. The various hard components of the earth provide structure and connection and are known as mineral or stone, the fourth element in the cosmological wheel.

Meanwhile, a steam of great density formed the atmosphere around the earth. (These images translate imperfectly into Western terms; think of them as poetic rather than scientific descriptions.) As the steam expanded, its pressure began to subside. The reduction of atmospheric pressure was conducive to the birth of life, and thus the fifth element, vegetative nature, came into being.

Life, as Dagara people say, began underwater. Thus, every living form on the earth got its life signature in the waters and continues to live intimately with water. It is as if the original encounter between fire and water established the conditions for life by producing a nurturing environment. Earth came to life as a result of the marriage between these two primal elements, and in turn Earth brought forth more life, which she continues to sustain. The idea that we all came from water is important because it implies that water is life, a concept we will return to later in the chapter.

As the pressure of the steam produced by the encounter of water and fire continued to subside, beings that were conceived in water looking like worms moved to dry land and continued to evolve. When the atmospheric pressure at last stabilized, the diversification of life slowed to an almost imperceptible state. Today, for instance, amphibious animals like crocodiles, sea lions, and seals are said to be beings that didn't complete their journey out of water. Their development was suspended when the atmospheric pressure stopped where it is today. On the other hand, beings who came out of the water earlier evolved into higher-dimensional spheres, allowing them to move back and forth in time and space. They embody our future. Birds are considered among the most ancient animals because they moved first from the water to the land, then continued to evolve to flight. Some elders say that, if things had continued to change, birds would have made it to other dimensions.

One might ask where this primal water came from. The elders, from their spiritual understanding, would say that it came from the Other World and spilled into the earth at a moment when the veil between the two worlds was thinned—the moment when the original Earth flew too close to the Other World. One might say that some kind of distortion occurred as the cool liquid Other World and the hot burning Earth passed too closely by each other. The distorted space sucked water out of the moist Other World and threw itself onto Earth. From this perspective, water is the presence of the Other World on our planet. The element fire is the doorway to the ancestors, but water is the doorway to the Other World, the kind of world that is referred to as the world of the *kontomblé* and the other nonancestral spirits. This is why shamans can walk into the Other World through the waterways. In fact there are countless places in water where these same veils still remain active. These veils are the umbilical cords, the gateways, linking our world to others.

The connection to the ancestral world that is found in the element fire is different from the connection with other beings and other intelligences. The spirits we call the *kontombli* and the spirits of the ancestors do not live in the same place, they don't share the same geography, yet they can communicate with each other. Just as here, the United States and Africa do not share the same geography, yet they can communicate, and there is communication going on all of the time. In an invocation, when you call to the spirits of your ancestors, and to the spirits of the elements, and to the helping spirits that you have some relationship with, you are calling on many many different worlds, and the connection to these worlds are through the elements of water and fire, which are the two worlds that are said to have come together originally to make Earth.

One might wonder how other worlds to which our world is linked were created. Indeed, the Dagara cosmology does not limit itself to this earth world but touches on others. This is because our world belongs to a family of worlds, without which it seems it cannot sustain itself. These Other Worlds were created in ways opposite to the way ours was created. In the creation stories, they came into being when their vast cool waters were hit by fire. The difference is that their vibration is much higher in intensity than the vibration of our world. This high-vibrational energy of the Other World permits the intelligence that lives in these worlds to come here easily. Apparently if the pressure of the atmosphere of our world had continued to evolve, it would have been easier for humans to journey into these worlds and back. Therefore spirituality—our efforts to enhance and advance our contact with the world of Spirit—is seen from an indigenous perspective as the continuation of human evolution.

EMBODYING THE FIVE ELEMENTS

People and cultures embody one or several of the five elements knowingly or not. The most commonly seen elements at the level of cultures are fire and water. Indigenous cultures identify with water. They are mostly peace and harmony seekers. On the contrary, modern cultures identify with fire. They challenge everything and everyone at the great risk of cosmic disruption.

Within these cultures, individuals are born embodying one of these elements as their essence and carrying the rest at a variety of levels as support elements. No one can be just one element without the presence of the other four. Your essence is your genius. Your destiny is to allow your genius to come out wrapped in the colors of your character. A person with vision and passion who is always active and involved in countless activities embodies fire. A person with a deep focus who tends to seek peaceful solution to conflicts, who always sees harmony instead of discord, embodies water. A person who tends to take care of others, accepting them as they are, embodies earth. A person with great social skills, who is always drawn to connect with others and who holds the stories of others, embodies mineral. Finally, a person who can't stand phoniness, who finds it impossible to pretend, who can only be himself or herself, embodies nature.

FIRE

Fire is the original element of origin, the one that was present at the beginning. Its primal nature is combustion, warmth, vision, and feeling. Its position in the wheel is the south, the underworld, and its color is red. It is the state to which everything eventually returns, the state the ancestors are in. As we walk the earth, we are warmed by the heat of the ancestors coming from the underworld below us. Fire opens the doorway to the

Spirit World and allows our psyche to commune with other life present, past, and future. Fire is like a connecting rod, an open channel. In fact, fire is our psyche, the spirit part of us that knows what has always been. It is our ability to act, emote, and intuit. A person on fire is craving a connection. In this person, fire is translated into restlessness, a great deal of emotion, and strong dream experience.

The fire person is someone with an eye to the world of the ancestors and the spirit. He or she is in charge of the gateway between this world and the other, the ancestral. This person understands dream imagery and can translate and interpret dream images to people. The fire person lives at the edge between human culture and ancestral culture. His or her task is to go back and forth between the two worlds. There is a unique aspect to such a person due to this ability to see into both worlds. Shamans fit into this category because they live in two worlds. They are not part of the common people, who fit well into their culture. They can see the culture from the perspective of the world of the spirit. Similarly, people who feel at the margins of their culture may be dealing with the fire of their culture. They cannot quite fit in, and other people have problems understanding why they won't behave like everybody else.

The fire person is often misunderstood by contemporaries because, with respect to this world, a fire person lives in the future and therefore finds the average person too slow. His or her behavior can be seen by the average person as impatient, hyperactive, and sometimes intolerant. A fire person cannot stay idle. However, his or her fire may be translated into a warm, gentle flame that keeps a whole village, community, town, or culture aware of its vital relationship with other worlds.

If a person or culture forgets its crucial relationship with other worlds, that is, with the ancestors, a fire is ignited that becomes a destructive force in society. When that happens, a person or a culture suddenly perceives almost everything in terms of fire. Fire becomes equated with power, speed, hierarchy, and value. All this is symptomatic of a culture in combustion. When one's culture is burning, it is impossible to sit still and keep focused. Like a ball of fire moving at high speed, a culture on fire is fascinated with speed. This speed shows up as horsepower on the surface, but deep within it is orchestrated by combustion. The burning within is symptomatic of some kind of crisis that drives people to remain endlessly "on fire."

The following description of a fiery culture may seem negative and unattractive. However, it is necessary to balance the positive elements of the fire person as an individual with the negative picture of a culture on fire. The reality is that fire is dangerous; when it runs out of control, it destroys everything in its path.

When a culture is caught in fire, its people's perception of the world is red. As they rush ceaselessly forward with a consumer's mentality, they pollute everything in their way, conquering and destroying anything that interferes. Fire culture promotes consumerism and cultivates scarcity in order to increase restlessness, then uses the restless, burning psyche as energy to increase production and consumption. Meanwhile the culture on fire is fascinated by violence. As a matter of fact, violence proves to be highly marketable and stimulates the fiery nature of the culture as a whole. Consequently, a fire culture is a war culture. It sees solutions in terms of fire and conflicts as fire that can be resolved with more fire. Such a culture will require a lot of water to heal.

WATER

We mentioned earlier that water encountered fire to produce the positive changes that generate life. The fiery earth was cooled and firmed, which allowed it to support life, and so became a whole realm to which water could now give life. We are in this story the children of water. Any person who understands the value of being the parent of a child knows that this is a great benefit. Water can claim us as her children. We can say that we come from Earth, but Earth didn't exist until water showed up, so water can lay claim to anything that is alive. Without water, nothing can be purified, nothing can be authentic. Water allows us to maintain the kind of consciousness that links us to the Other World, and hence we see in so many mythologies the idea of water as the "water of life," with water crucial to the spiritual experience and the spiritual journey.

The element water reconciles and quiets down that which is trapped in the crisis of combustion. In effect, water cools the burning psyche. It stills the restless consciousness and bestows serenity upon a person in turmoil, returning focus to a chaotic existence. As an elemental unit in the cosmological wheel, its position is the north, opposite fire, and its colors are blue and black. Water seeks to cleanse, reconcile, and balance that which is in agitation, emotional disorder, and self-danger. When water succeeds, it restores or enhances life where there was the threat of death. Hence the connection between water and life. To seek water is to seek to reconcile and balance that which is constantly in danger of being thrown out of balance, that which is caught in the fiery loop of speed and consumption.

To seek water is to seek the vitality and blossoming that comes from successful self-immersion. Water encourages a positive slowdown that permits one to notice things that are usually overlooked at high speed, and for this reason water is associated with focus. The water person is slow, shows great understanding, and is eager to make things work for the greatest good. He or she perceives the world in terms of possibilities. The water person thinks of community, relationship, love, and harmony. Water is therefore also grief. Among other causes, grief arises from recognizing the loss that occurs from our failure to notice, and grief comes also from recognizing the wide gap between what is possible and the impossibility of getting there. The salted taste of tears of grief is the cleansing taste of reconciliation, of the desire to reconcile, because water cleanses and washes away the impurities of our failures. Grief is the enemy of denial. An elder once told me, "My tears say that my soul has heard something about the Other World."

When the world is out of balance and unreconciled, the waters are polluted, mistreated. They become the dumping ground of the world's ignominies. So pollution is not a sign of progress. It is the sign of crisis and the inability to reconcile. Pollution is the exhaust system of human denial. The disabled water lies useless while humans in the midst of fire speed along their way looking for a means of reconciliation. Meanwhile, life-sustaining water must be rationed in many areas. It is as if fire doesn't like the presence of water.

A water culture likes to keep things the way they are. Such a culture does not want the natural and environmental harmony to be perturbed. It is a slow culture with very little temper. It prefers to see the potential good in anything. People who have too much water have little ambition. They are not in a hurry to do or to complete anything. They perceive time very broadly and are annoyed when they are compelled to hurry up. They think about all the things they never accomplish, and if they are badly out of balance in the direction of water, they do not even have regrets about them.

EARTH

Earth symbolizes the mother on whose lap everyone finds a home, nourishment, support, comfort, and empowerment. Representing the principle of inclusion, earth is the ground upon which we identify ourselves and others. It is what gives us identity and a sense of belonging. Produced as the result of the encounter between fire and water, earth represents survival and healing, unconditional love and caring. Earth loves to give and gives love abundantly. In other words, earth cares as much for the crooked as it does for the honest. Both of them are allowed to walk on her. In the Dagara cosmological wheel, earth is located in the center and is colored yellow. This central position in the wheel stresses the importance of visibility. Earth is the power to notice, to see and to thrill in being seen.

The person who is of earth is a lover of the world, of the earth. Unlike water, which seeks a way always toward one place, the ocean, earth finds comfort everywhere, anywhere, and loves to give it. Earth people, or people with a lot of earth energy, are nurturers who, like all grandmothers, want everybody to feel fed, content, respected, and loved. Earth people can't stand the presence of scarcity; they would give away everything they had before they gave anything to themselves. Making others feel good makes them feel good. The earth person takes care of other people spiritually, materially, and emotionally.

A person without earth is in crisis, or is homeless and in exile. Such a person has lost his or her grounding. A person without earth feels empty, alone, and confused. She or he suffers from invisibility and anonymity. This unbearable situation can cause a whole culture to sell homes or parcels of earth to each other. This is because home in the symbolic or literal sense is the basic ground for identity. If you remove people's home from them and then offer it to them for sale, people will have to buy it, because being homeless is unendurable. Thus pieces of our mother have entered into our trade system with great success. Is this why Western culture feels odd in front of homelessness? Is it why it doesn't know what to do with those people who can't fit economic expectations? Land and the earth are now a commodity, and this fact will not change.

My point here is that the development of industrial economies and the movement of vast numbers of people into the cities has not changed the essential connection between human beings and the earth that engendered them; it has only caused them to forget. When the people of a culture no longer remember that they are but a thread of the web of life on Earth, then they all become homeless.

Building community is difficult, if not impossible, if people have lost contact with the ground as their point of strength. For it is only from a place of grounding and centeredness that anyone can give something back to their world, to their community. Without grounding people will tend to take as much from the world as possible, since they are missing the nourishment that earth offers. Yet after they have gained all the material things they need, they will still feel uncertain about themselves. It indicates that they have not yet felt invited to give something to the world. To take without prior giving is like putting the cart ahead of the horse. You are not grounded. Deep down you do not know where you come from, and therefore you are unsure about where you are going and why. Earth, the spiritual shrine of our being, is the center of being deeply human.

BUILDING A HOME

Because Earth is our deep center, it is the center of rituals concerning the building of a home. It is appropriate to dwell on the ritual of house building among Dagara people, to highlight its relevance to community and the sense of belonging. Among the Dagara, because the house is the most visible symbol of the earth, home is sacred. Similarly there is a link between home and relationships, especially the relationship between the family and the community. This is why building a home is a very serious ritual undertaking. It is as if building a house is building a relationship.

According to Dagara custom, men build the structure of houses, and women make them come alive. Before a man builds a home, he must bring a gift of fifteen hundred cowrie shells and a chicken to the village's earth shrine. The cowrie shells represent abundance, the chicken represents life. The priest of the earth shrine takes the gift from the prospective homeowner and presents it to the earth spirit mother with a prayer of support. This prayer of support often takes the form of an invocation to the earth spirit to assist in the birthing of a new family. Then both the priest and the prospective homeowner strike the ground together with the same hoe. This gesture of cracking the ground open is symbolic of planting one's roots, even though it is not the place where the new home is built.

After this the prospective homeowner notifies the priest of the ancestors' shrine, who is usually the chief of the village, of his intention to build. The next ritual will take place at the building location and will involve the priest of the ancestors' shrine and include, once again, the scratching of the ground while praying for community. The prayer translates roughly as, "This is the expression of a desire to come together, not to part together." To form a community requires the blessing of the ancestors if it will sprout and grow.

From then onward the house is built by stages, each of which is ritualized with sacrifices and offerings to the spirit of the ground and to the ancestors. All of this takes months to complete. The section of the home for
animals is built first, because of the respect due to animals. Almost at the
same time as the animal section is finished, a roof is placed over a small
section intended for people. A home becomes a home when it has a roof,
for at that moment the spirits that support the family move in. Someone of
the family must move in immediately, to keep the supportive spirits from
leaving, for an unoccupied house invites evil spirits. Soon after the roof is
put in place, the women's quarters are completed, and the women and
children move in. No bathroom is built into the house, since people use
nature for sanitation, and human waste fertilizes the farmland. The man
of the house will be the last one to move into the new home.

People occupy the new house, but the true owner is considered to be
Tingan, the spirit of the earth. Because Tingan owns the home, every
household problem is a message from Tingan, including sickness and re-
lational crises. When such a crisis occurs, it is the result of a distancing
from Tingan, and family members must consult a diviner to find out what
Tingan wants.

The home is a direct extension of the relationship between members
of a family and the village. The breaking of the new ground must, therefore, be undertaken with the presence of the community. The gradual
move is made necessary because the process of shifting the location of the
relationship is a delicate one. The extensive set of rituals serves the purpose of allowing the existing relationship between the family and the
community to be transferred safely to a new location, a new ground.

There is no move-in ritual, because the move does not take place the
day you change location, but the day you think about changing location.
In this case, the ritual done with the priests of the earth shrine and the ancestors at the beginning of the process can be considered the move-in rituals.

MINERAL OR STONE

From the element earth we move to the fourth element, mineral. Mineral is the storage place of memory, the principle of creativity, resources, stories, and symbolism. In the cosmological wheel, mineral is located in the west and is colored white. It is the elemental energy that allows us to remember, to communicate with one another, to express our feelings, to receive messages from the Other World, and to remember our origins and purpose in this life. These functions are what the human skeletal structure, made of mineral, is all about. In Dagara physiology, our bones, not the brain, are the storage place of memory. In the village it is not uncommon to hear an elder say, "This is in our bones as it was in the bones of our ancestors." In the West there is a similar saying, "I knew it in my bones," which refers to a deeper, more elemental knowing than is possible through rational thought.

To the indigenous person, mineral is also equivalent to stone. As they say, the bones of the earth are the stones and rocks we see. To know the true story of our earth, including the story of ourselves, is to listen to the rocks. They are the conduits through which earth passes information on to us. Any creature that is born with bones is said to be born already possessing some knowledge. This is where the indigenous derive their belief that no one comes into this world without a genius, and that this genius must be opened to the person shortly after birth, first through the name, and later on through initiation. All those in Western culture who wander without purpose are perhaps stripped of their genius and are in exile searching for ways to remember. These are people in need of mineral rituals, to repair their relationship to memory, which is symbolized in mineral.

Indigenous people think that our bones are the minerals in which we store thousands of years of information. They store that which we need to remember. This makes me wonder if many problems of the West are a result of forgetting. I wonder also if those in Silicon Valley who shave stones to their essence and put them in machines of memory perhaps already know somehow that stones have always managed information. My sense is that those who experience midlife crises are responding to the pull and push of masses of information they have not been using because they can't fully remember. For example, if there were a way to help people use the deep memories that they brought with them into this life, it would make a tremendous difference in their sense of direction and purpose.

I wonder also if part of the modern world's fascination with the Internet can be traced to this vast memory gap. People are searching for something, and when the information stored in our bones is neglected, one feels the urge to go outside the self in search of it. If the information out there echoes the information inside of us, could it be that the great turmoil of unrecognized wisdom within us is forcing us to race along the information superhighway, hoping that we will discover what we already have? The proliferation of various software to make the venture even easier would support this thought: does Windows 95 suggest the promise of a peek into the Other World?

Indigenous people don't learn by looking outside themselves; instead, they learn how to remember the knowledge they already possess. The person who has a mineral nature speaks a great deal because mineral expresses in discourse what is stored in coded form within the bones.

Mineral people are storytellers, fascinated with myth, tradition, and rituals, versed in dealing with metaphors and symbols. In Africa, they are the town criers who know what happens now and what has happened for countless generations. They constantly remind us in stories, proverbs, songs, and poems the deep healing significance of staying connected. They know how to praise and how to warn.

A culture weighted too heavily with mineral is frenetically involved with communication at every level. In such a culture, language is an impressive instrument of power. The problem with such a culture is in finding an audience, or someone to listen. A mineral person's love for argument, for different ways of saying the same thing, and for eloquent ways of saying nothing can baffle the nonmineral person. In truth, a mineral person or culture is extroverted, almost bombastic, but almost always has a point. The gift they present to their society and the world is the gift of remembering, through words and stories, one's origins and purpose.

NATURE

The element of nature signifies the principle of change. It is transformation, mutation, adjustment, flexibility, cyclicality, life, death, and magic. Nature is vegetative, therefore it is all plants and landscapes; and it is all animals as well. In the cosmological wheel nature is situated in the east, opposite mineral, and its color is green. Nature invites us to change consciously and to welcome change. Just as mineral stores information for our benefit, nature's complex paradigm is a library to those who pay attention. The magic we crave and our attraction to the supernatural are nature in their essence. This is because the tree, the plant, the landscape, and the serpentine river zigzagging downhill on its way to the ocean are all golden hieroglyphs capable of bringing a deep understanding to those willing to pay attention. Indeed, to the indigenous it seems that the tree is the essence of consciousness.

Landscapes and physical geography to indigenous people are a language, a writing that can be read. Elevated areas function very much like antennae, relaying or downloading information from faraway places, from the outer world to the inner world. Waterways take this information down to the underworld and carry messengers to the underworld.

Barren and flat landscapes emit a fast-moving energy that is dangerous to isolated individuals. The Dagara see a desert as a place where faraway beings meet day and night. During the day they are not busy and the light hides them, but at night they are active and much more visible. Since one can get caught in their world and never find one's way back, only medicine men and women venture into wide open places at night.

In heavily forested areas the moisture of nature and the trees protects and shields human beings from the Other World. But at the same time, because the tall trees are engaged in some mysterious activities, especially at night, normal people should not be exposed to them, for they emit an energy that could affect their psyches as well as their bodies. This leaves the ideal living place, for the Dagara, as the savanna, with its sparse trees and tall grass. Because such a place is sandwiched between two highly charged geographies, it is a refuge for human beings.

Every life form is touched by this galactic communications system located in the geography. This is why unlike in the West, where nature and magic are often opposed, the indigenous see the two as inseparable.

The nature person is seen as a person with great power to adjust, to change shape and shift. He or she is a witch, a magician. I have often wondered if the Puritans did not destroy witches because of their fear of the great power of nature within them. Western history is full of persecution of the natural and of nature. Today, even if witches are no longer burned alive, it remains that nature itself is being destroyed. Every time a tree is felled, another witch is terminated. Every time a place is cleared by a developer, a magical gift from the earth is crushed. Progress seems to point to nature as its main enemy. Justified by economics, it acts in disgust toward nature, as if nature were standing in its way.

Nature people challenge us to be real, to be ourselves. They challenge us to drop the mask that the world expects us to wear, and they challenge us to see what is around us as it truly is. That challenge comes in the form of humor, play, and joy, which has tremendous subversive power. Nature people trick us through humor and jokes into being real. A nature person is like a child who loves to play and sees life as a challenging play. In such a person, pretense is hard to come by. The power of nature is not just in its magical abilities, but also in the kind of change it pushes us to make.

For this reason, a culture dominated by nature will be extremely sensitive to the cycles of life. Its spirituality will be dominated by seasonal rituals to keep time with the changing rhythm of nature. The mythology and stories of such a culture will be crowded with trees and animals that speak, with beings that live underneath the waterways and inside mountains and hills. The people will tend to see living spirits behind birds,

trees, and other animals, and will have complicated protocols for interacting with them. In the indigenous world, this is so true that an outsider may
wonder how people manage to live with this consciousness. The shadow
side of nature is black magic, the kind that is believed to harm other
people. This is why even though a witch is not a black magician, he or she
is feared because of knowing how such magic works.

It is my sense that if incorporating any of these five elements poses a
challenge to modernity, then the challenge posed by nature is the most difficult of all. Indigenous people think that to be modern requires a move
away from nature. They can't see how nature can be combined with
modernity, for modern technology sets itself up in opposition to nature.
But indigenous people also know that nature does not make compromises.
It does not flinch when confronted, because its own destruction means our
destruction. For this reason, indigenous people embrace the wisdom of
living close to nature and respecting its wishes.

THE FIVE ELEMENTS AND COMMUNITY

I have been using names such as water people, fire people, earth people,
mineral people, and nature people. Indeed, these five elements are also de-
finable by clan; people are born into one or another of the clans, much like
being born under a certain astrological sign. It is the time of your birth
that stamps the element it carries on you. The decision of when to be born
and therefore which element to embody is considered by indigenous
people to be prenatal and is sealed by the individual.

The five elements, which make up five clans, together allow the entire
village to form a cosmological wheel. The village can then balance itself
by keeping the various elements in balance. For the wheel to be balanced,
there must be an overwhelming representation of water. Just as the earth
is essentially water, and just as the human body is essentially water, a community needs a large number of water people to maintain its balance.
There must be at least three times more people of water in the village than

people of fire. When there are not, symbolic heat creeps in and rises, resulting in crisis. The difficulty of forming community in the modern world seems to arise from this, for when the people coming together are predominantly of fire, friction is produced more often than balance.

This is why there are healing rituals aimed at coping with problems of imbalance. Water rituals can help calm the fire and produce reconciliation with nature. Indeed, when the proportion of water is more than three times that of fire, the earth becomes moist enough for nature to flourish. Water feeds nature, so the presence of water results in a vitally growing plant and animal life. A healthy relationship of water, earth, and nature will result in clean air to breathe. When these three elements are not in balance, the air we breathe is poor in quality. To upset the balance of elements is to throw the community into danger.

The principal task of a community is to maintain balance, a state in which all five elements are functioning smoothly, echoing one another. To achieve this requires great diligence on the part of a community. This effort need not be undertaken through the application of sophisticated theories of economics or social welfare. It is first necessary to determine which elements are troubling the community. We will have ample space to explore this in the chapters devoted to the elements and ritual. It is sufficient for now to know that there is an elemental way of understanding social and economic problems, and that there is a way to resolve these problems through ritual.

The elemental wheel exists in each person just as it is present in each clan and in every community. This means that each person, on a smaller scale, must maintain a state of balance at all cost. Each person needs to keep the waters of reconciliation flowing within the self, in order to calm the inner fires and live in harmony with others. Each person needs to nourish the ancestral fire within, so that one stays in touch with one's dreams and visions. Each person needs to be grounded in the earth, to be able to become a source of nourishment to the community. Each person needs to remember the knowledge stored in one's bones—to live out one's own unique genius. And each person needs to be real, as nature is real, that is, without pretense, keeping in touch with a sense of mystery and wonder and helping to preserve the integrity of the natural world. To be out of balance in any of these areas is to invite sickness to come dwell within.

A person who is out of balance threatens to throw the entire community out of balance. In the village, the illness of any one person calls forth the energy of the entire community. If any individual is sick, then the village is sick. A community is healthy when everybody in it is healthy. The fire of a person who is in an emotional crisis can easily expand out to other people and before the problem is identified, the entire community could be ablaze.

In the modern world ideological or dogmatic thought can be quite dangerous in a similar way. Ideology and dogma contain an elemental fiery energy of a distinct signature that can surge. Without protective efforts, the surging energy can spread to other circuits and enflame a whole system, a whole culture. Individual healing can be seen as a protection of life's energetic wheel, for only when all of the individuals in a community are healthy can there be health in the community itself.

THE FIVE ELEMENTS AND RITUAL

Ritual is for the purpose of restoring balance, the essence of health, to individual and community. It serves no purpose to know the functional meaning of these cosmological elements if the ultimate reason is unconnected to ritual. To the extent that ritual is born out of the understanding of the cosmological wheel, the elements are its molecular tools whose proportion to one another must be monitored and restored when needed. The procedure for this is ritual. Fire rituals rekindle the connection to the ancestral fire and the fire within with vision. Water rituals cleanse and reconcile, restoring peace. Earth rituals ground and comfort, bringing a sense of home and belonging. Mineral rituals restore memory and light up a sense of knowing. Nature rituals restore the natural self and open us up to the magic and wonder around us.

When a group of people gathers to conduct a ritual, in an indigenous context, people who embody each of the elements become the gatekeepers for that particular element in the ritual and for the part of the ritual pertaining to that element. As we saw in chapter 2, a gatekeeper is a healer who by his or her nature is able to bridge this world and the Other World, allowing the healing gifts from the world of Spirit to be brought into the physical world. The gatekeepers of each element are those people whose genius, whose essential character, embodies the gifts of that element. By virtue of the fact that you carry a certain gift, you are given a special relationship with the element from which that gift originated, and in this sense you are a gatekeeper. You stand between the rest of the community and that portion of the natural world that corresponds to your element and all that it represents symbolically.

For instance, the gift of a person with the power to make people dream, or to awaken their intuitive and emotional selves, is associated with a gateway connected to fire. The gift that a person has of bringing a sense of peace and completeness and focus to others is associated with a gateway connected to water. The gift that a person has to nurture and support and accept others is associated with a gateway connected to the earth. The gift that a person has of producing meaningful images in the mind of another, allowing people to remember in a flash of insight, is associated with a gateway connected to the stones or what we call mineral. The gift that a person has of allowing other people to be real, to just be themselves without reservation, is associated with a gateway connected to nature.

A person's gifts, when they emerge, make the carrier of the gift a servant to a particular gate, and because they are the servant to that particular gate, we call them gatekeepers. Though every person embodies one element in particular, all elements must be present in each person.

The Dagara people have developed this notion of gatekeeping, of overseeing something vital to the healthy functioning of the community, in order to support and satisfy people's innate desire to serve. By serving the gateway to an elemental aspect of the natural world, a person allows the qualities and resources that element represents to be brought to the community, giving the community what it needs to blossom fully.

In the rituals outlined in the following chapters, suggestions are made for roles that gatekeepers can play in serving the community by serving the shrine of their particular element. Since part of the work of ritual is to prepare the space for the ritual, and since much of the work of preparing the space is done through building a shrine to the element on which the ritual focuses, a few words on shrine building are in order.

BUILDING SHRINES

Shrines at their simplest define a space where the work of ritual can occur. In the presence of shrines, it is easy to engage in ritual. Shrines incorporate natural elements to remind us that this is a space different from our everyday world, inviting us to undertake something different from our everyday work. They create a space that, when we step into it, invites us for a while to forget time and the mundane world so that we can focus on our deeper selves and on the timeless realities that can be seen in the natural world that surrounds us. They remind us of the mystery that exists in the world, of those things that are still unknown.

What takes the place of community shrines in the West are often only monuments that refer to past violence or the threat of violence suppressed by the glory of victory. For example, monuments of war, military symbols, and nationalist emblems become substitutes for real shrines. I must make an exception here of the Vietnam Veterans' Memorial in Washington, D.C., which would be seen indigenously as a true shrine. Similarly the statue of Abraham Lincoln at his memorial, radiating compassion and sadness, points to the sacred. But even these powerful shrines point out another problem with Western shrines. They are often concerned with history, whereas indigenous shrines ignore time altogether.

I have learned that people in the West do know how to make shrines. Time and again, I have had the opportunity to guide Western men and women in building shrines, and in most cases it has been a success. Each has managed to incorporate some of the most important features of a shrine, including beauty and mystery. The builders needed to understand that a shrine must be made of natural things, picked from the natural world. They also needed to trust in their imagination, following the basic warning that their imagination must reject such industrial products as aluminum foil, plastic, and artificial decorations.

Shrines, especially shrines built in nature, are designed to blend with their natural surroundings. A large part of the shrine for any element is on the earth, for the earth touches all of the other elements. Shrines are never intended to tower over or dominate the natural world. The entry to the shrine must be obvious to an observer, and often arching branches serve to mark clearly the gateway that separates the sacred space of the shrine from the mundane world. Symbolic items, preferably hand-made such as necklaces, amulets, stones, or statues that hold some significance for the individuals that will participate in the ritual, are a type of decoration that brings a useful focus to the work that is to be done at the shrine. In the workshops I do with people in the West, there are usually no props provided when shrines are built, only the broadest outlines, as I have described above. The reason is simple: it is not healthy to provide a finished product to a group of people, because a shrine must reflect the state of imagination of the people who build it. The many successful shrines that have been built prove to me that in the West, as in an indigenous village, there is an innate understanding about the nature of sacred space.

At a typical workshop, which focused on the reconnection with the five elements described above, people were divided into five groups according to the elements they embodied. Fire people built a shrine by gathering together red cloth and objects that reminded them of the energy of fire, such as statues or photos of departed ones—some even brought the ashes of their departed ones—and a lot of red stones. They rounded up votive candles and placed them on an impromptu pedestal made of boxes.

When all the candles were lit, the whole thing looked like a burning stairway leaping up from the underground and rising into the sky.

Water people took the colors blue and black and created a shrine that flowed out of one corner of the room like a waterway. A black shawl flowed between two large bowls of water. A few candles were floating inside the bowls of water, while other candles, blue and black, decorated the shrine. When one looked at it, the sense of flow was obvious. On the shrine, they placed their personal objects of power, such as photos of water gods and goddesses, carvings of fish, and shells.

Earth people brought in a pile of dirt and made a big mound out of it. It was held in place by large rocks. On it they planted what looked like trees against a yellow cloth background. The top of the mound was curved like a lap to give a sense of the loving mother. Around it they placed various statues made with clay and representing the mother. It was big enough for a person to sit on. The whole shrine was lit with yellow candles.

Mineral people hauled in a great number of rocks and built a kind of grotto out of it. The grotto was protected by branches and leaves. On the rocks they placed white candles that when lit made the shrine look like the burning bush. They too had power objects placed on their shrine. These power objects were mostly a large variety of stones.

Finally, nature people recreated a sense of the jungle with greens picked up from the surrounding outdoors. They cropped treelike shapes, which they then brought alive with a lot of green. A few green candles were placed carefully so that they could be seen only when lit.

Once people have chosen the element around which to build their ritual and their shrine, and once the space has been prepared, chances are that some inner preparation for ritual has also been done. But preparing one's psyche for ritual is so important that to it we now turn.

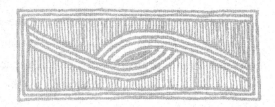

9.

Preparing for Ritual

It is a long long way
If you listen to your mind
It is a short short way
If you listen to your heart
—MIRKO UDZENIJA

Most of the rituals that follow in Part Four can be performed by Westerners as described and, with a little imagination, can be modified and expanded to fit many specific situations. But in order for healing to take place, careful attention must be given to the conscious and unconscious attitudes carried by the participants. One of the most striking things that I have observed in conducting rituals with people in the West is the overwhelming baggage of assumptions that stand in the way of their involvement with ritual. Among these problems are the need for predictability and control and a fear of what is actually going to happen. Reverence and trust that there is protection in the sacred space and an open mind willing to embrace all possibilities for healing are necessary before any ritual begins.

Almost everyone who has been involved in ritual with me agrees that ritual is like a journey. Before you begin, you own the journey; once the ritual begins, the journey owns you. My sense is that at the core of the problem for many Westerners is the desire to be in control, which is antithetical to ritual. To surrender the sense of control can be, for some, terrifying.

RITUAL FROM BELOW

Anthropologist Victor Turner has given us an instructive picture of the difference between indigenous and modern approaches to ritual. In *The Ritual Process* he refers to ascending symbolism as opposed to descending symbolism in order to clarify the distinction between indigenous ritual practices and Western ceremonial practices.

The Western view of authority as something that comes from above dramatically affects one's perception of the source of transformation and change. The assumption is that if anything transcendental is going to happen, it has to come from above and descend to humans. Ever since Christianity unearthed the gods and goddesses and sent them far away above the clouds, many people in the West have been left standing on the ground feeling abandoned, staring longingly at the sky wondering when God will come. In contrast, indigenous people see the divine as arising from below. Indeed, the ancestors, who dwell under the earth and form a vast pool of energy, allow us to walk upon them. Thus the divine is right under our feet and directly connected to us through the earth. This perception calls for a significantly different attitude that encourages spontaneity and trust of one's instincts, because it sees redemption and healing as rising like heat from the divine below. Ritual therefore follows an ascending principle, presuming that healing rises from under the earth and overtakes us.

In this context, spontaneity, improvisation, and even eccentricity are recognized as symptomatic of divine presence. No one can predict how an individual in whom Spirit has entered would behave, because no one really knows the behavioral psychology of Spirit. Therefore to expect attitudes and behavior patterns similar to that with which we are familiar is misleading. In rituals people are expected to respond to the challenge of Spirit and to surrender to something bursting up from beneath their feet. Because this bursting is unpredictable and cannot be repeated twice— since Spirit never moves the same person the same way—the indigenous believe that a ritual happens only once and is never repeated again. What makes it work is the Spirit that is invited into it, and Spirit rarely repeats what it has done.

Put simply, rituals are not, and cannot be, done mechanically. They require a level of involvement that is conscious and dynamic. It is the active participation of the people gathered that makes a ritual work. In part this means that one can't approach ritual in an experimental or exploratory manner, for it may backfire on you. It also means that it is better not to do ritual at all than to do it badly. A bad ritual is one that resists the arrival of Spirit. It is one in which participants allow their own desires and preconceptions to compete with Spirit, particularly after inviting Spirit to come.

RITUAL AND SURRENDER

Participants need to understand that success in a ritual is proportional to the level of surrender that one can achieve. Because ritual is about change, its success depends on how much change, and what change, if any, we are willing to invite. Modern culture is a culture of control. You are expected to be on top of things, to take control and to show your command of it. The result is often disastrous to the psyche. On the one hand, people show admirable dexterity in appearing cool. On the other hand, behind the sturdy look of a person perfectly in charge is often a soul adrift in a jungle of confusion and despair. A soul in despair is a soul denying access to Spirit. A soul that dances with Spirit is a soul that has displaced ego and, in the interest of healing, has surrendered consciousness to Spirit.

Surrender is a difficult thing to achieve; it is almost impossible to do it with words and discourse. The more the discussion about how to do ritual emphasizes surrender and letting go, the more conscious and unconscious resistance one generates. I have seen cases in which it took three days of painful and frustrating work to prepare people to truly attempt a ritual. This preparatory stage is most challenging because it opens potent issues of self-identity, integrity, protectiveness, and control. As people begin to understand what ritual is, they realize that their own ego has no place in it, that sacred space contains a tremendous amount of vulnerability. Then they begin to fear becoming lost in something that does not guarantee safety and security.

The latent mistrust of one another that exists among people does not help. In fact it makes people become more acutely aware of what the other may do to them if they lower their shield in the interest of healing and the other does not. In most ritual situations in the West, people have just met and have only had a few hours or days to get acquainted. The connection that develops in a few hours or a few days often does not go as deep as required to warrant the kind of trust that can carry people into a ritual space and promote healing.

But once inside a ritual, the ego is so vehemently challenged that it eventually collapses, leaving a person momentarily free to respond to Spirit spontaneously. I have, at times, been so shocked by this sudden surrender that at first I refused to believe what my eyes were seeing. I remember in particular one man who, as we talked about an earth ritual, was terribly nervous and showed it by the kind of questions he was asking. First we talked about walking to a pit and entering it, and he wondered which foot to move first. Then he asked if he should enter the earth hole with his legs or with his head. Then he admitted that the ritual did not make sense at all. When the actual ritual began, the man took on the posture of an observer. When he saw how deeply involved others were, he loosened up. Something like a wild energy burst out of him. He began dancing and chanting very loudly, even clapping his hands. When his turn came to go to the earth, he was the humblest of all. Later he said to everyone that he had found his new drug, and it is ritual.

From this, however, I have learned that every human being, including the most educated and sophisticated, desires ritual almost more than anything else. They want it for the resuscitation of the wild and wise savage who hides somewhere in the psychic recesses of even the most highly cultured person. They want it because of the eternal craving of that part of the self that will never quit wanting to be intimate with Spirit. This is perhaps why indigenous people cannot separate themselves from rituals.

In the modern world, however, the absence of ritual has led to more destructive ritualistic behaviors like drug and alcohol abuse, and the attraction to violence and sex. Indigenous people have made ritual central in their lives because it takes care of their needs at the deepest level. In ritual, the world of peace and transcendence sought by the person who is addicted to drugs and alcohol is reached without damage to the body. Colonial invaders broke down indigenous culture by replacing healthy ritual with alcohol. A principal reason why the remaining indigenous world is currently suffering in the grip of an epidemic of alcoholism is that alcohol has removed and replaced healthy ritual. For this reason also it is difficult to do anything pertaining to ritual in the modern world, where destructive addictions occupy the place normally reserved for rituals.

PERSONAL RITUALS

In the West more than anywhere else, the lack of community has increased the need for personal rituals. Personal rituals are generally done to keep oneself in harmony with the surrounding world. Personal rituals are for the most part maintenance rituals. In them, one cultivates and maintains an awareness of an affinity with the Spirit World in the form of an ancestor, or in some physical spirit, such as a bird or other animal-shaped entity. Among the most urgently needed personal rituals are rituals to heal one's connection with the ancestors and to heal the ancestors themselves, rituals to commune with spirit allies that are waiting to become more active in our lives, and basic self-maintenance rituals.

My younger sister provides an example of being moved to do personal rituals on behalf of ancestors and spirit allies. She used to tell me about dreams of an almost unbelievable nature filled with trees dripping with fruits. I thought she was compensating in her dreams for the scarcity of rain and the ongoing drought plaguing the tribal lands. But she told the dreams with such an insistence that in the end I had to accept the plain reality of her dream world. She would wake up in the middle of the night, forced out of her sleep by a loud noise, to find herself in a golden place crowded with shining people moving from one place to another without having to move their legs.

These small golden people were mostly friendly. They had a message for her having to do with a ritual. One of them held a bright white chicken in one hand and had three fingers outstretched. Another one held a white piece of cloth and a golden crown. A third one sat near the family shrine with a clay pot full of water. After being shown all these ritual objects, she would watch our maternal aunt, who had been dead for nearly twenty years, walk into the room laden with expensive costumes and jewelry.

My sister said she would try to get up and get away from our aunt because she knew she was dead. But she could not, and, as if the spirit knew her fear and desire to flee, our aunt would smile at her and stretch her hand out to her in a maternal way. But as she reached out to grab the loving hand, everything would disappear with a loud noise. The next voice she would hear would be her father in-law, asking her what was happening. As she began to answer him, she would realize that no one but she had seen what had taken place.

Eventually my sister learned that certain spirit allies had befriended her the moment she was born and were following her. In her dream they were trying to tell her what ritual she should do in order for her life to change for the good. Although it took her a few years to understand what she had been asked to do, she finally became aware of these spirits in her day-to-day life. Each time she calls on them now they respond. She is the only one that can hear them, and she can ask them anything and they will answer. To maintain and feed the connection to these spirits that have personally befriended her requires a dedicated and ongoing ritual practice by my sister. This is an example of personal rituals involving ancestors and spirit allies.

Ancestor rituals help to heal the ancestors themselves and our connections with them. Ancestors are those who reside in the Spirit World through the loss of their physical bodies. The West is full of horror stories about those who perpetrate abuses from beyond the grave. Part of this tradition comes from the fact that those who die after living an unclean life become suddenly aware of what they have done and desperately seek cooperation from the living in order to heal. As a result, it is not difficult to notice that among families where a death is recently experienced, some are able to go on with life as if nothing happened, while others remain perpetually uneasy and troubled.

Those who are knowledgeable will see in almost every family at least one person who functions as the receptacle of energies from the Other World, one family member who has the sensitivity to be aware of, and respond to, the deeper spiritual and sometimes physical needs of the family across generations. Sometimes these people are recognized as caretakers of the family. They are called on for every need any family member has, and, in some cases, blamed for problems that the family encounters. The life of these people is not easy. Often they see things that are very disturbing, including visions of departed loved ones. In the worst scenarios, they are deeply disturbed and worried about serious wrongs throughout the culture. They feel danger all around them.

In the indigenous world, these people are the shamans, the shrine keepers, and the healers of the family tree. They are being hailed by family members and friends in this world, and by departed ancestors from the

Other World who need healing. In this situation, the first thing they must do is to build an altar to the dead. Preferably, the shrine will have a lot of red in it to represent fire, which is symbolic of the ancestors, and will carry pictures of the departed ones. There should always be some food samples on the shrine constantly replenished to maintain their freshness.

They should go to the shrine every evening, perhaps also every morning, to spend time speaking to the ancestors. The most important time is spent there at night, prior to going to bed. Because the dead don't hesitate to come into dreams, it is important to let them know that one is willing to take whatever steps are necessary to normalize the relationship with them and to help heal them. The ancestors must have clear instructions and should be invited to come in a dream. Ancestors usually love directions like this. The line between this side and the other side is not such that things coming to us from there are always clear and understandable. We must help our needy ancestors learn to communicate with us. Otherwise they think we understand and have simply chosen not to reply or comply.

In the indigenous world dissatisfied ancestors are believed to be the instigators of violent death. A culture in which people die accidentally is said to have a dysfunctional relationship with its ancestors. It is the ancestors' way of attracting attention to something crucial to everyone's wellbeing. You know that the ancestors are healed when things begin to change dramatically for the better around you. The healed ancestors will bring health, prosperity, and a sense of intimate connection that is unparalleled.

Ancestors are at a disadvantage because they know how to improve things and yet they do not have the body required to act on what they know. We are at a disadvantage because, although we have bodies, we often lack the knowledge required to carry things out properly. This is why Spirit likes to work through us. A person with a body is an ideal vehicle for Spirit to manifest things in this world. It is important to understand that when we feel that something is missing in our life, when we feel somehow disconnected or displaced, that these feelings are a sign for us to repair our connection with the world of the ancestors and spirits.

Another form of personal ritual is that which honors and develops our connections to spirit allies. We are surrounded by allies of which we make little use. In a culture that honors self-reliance, the tendency is to take on the world alone and to feel personally weak in the face of failure. We respond to the cultural message that says we are alone in the universe and that ultimately nothing exists there to support us. We are asked to believe in a God that is very high up, so high up that one must live as if this life here does not count very much. At best we live a life that can only take advantage of the little pleasure that comes near us, only to find ourselves wanting more depth.

In an attempt to let us know that, in truth, we are not alone, countless spirits call upon us from the depth of our bones. They keep coming up with new ways to get our attention. These are what we call our spirit allies. They have been with us before, and continue to be with us, but they want a relationship with us in which we give as well as take. The further we distance ourselves from them, the more destruction we create or encounter around us. The closer we are to them, or the more responsive we are, the more healing they make available to us.

There is no one right or wrong way to respond to the call of Spirit. The important thing is that we talk to them. Even if we just tell them that we don't have time to talk or that we're too busy trying to pay bills, this reciprocation is a start in the right direction. Through even the most informal personal ritual, our initial responses deepen into a realization of what we've been missing by taking on the whole world alone. We come to understand that our sense of belonging in this world is proportional to our sense of continuity with the Other World.

In the indigenous mind, a person in trouble in this world was already in trouble in the Other World. So the first thing to do is to get out of trouble in the Other World. This is why ritual exists.

If we feel out of touch, it may very well be a reflection of a widespread disassociation, or the fact that important links with the Other World are loosening. Self-maintenance rituals are personal rituals based on the need to maintain and monitor our state of connectedness. They require that we be able to hear well, and notice the smallest signs around us, the softest messages directed at us. Noticing is more important than understanding what you notice. From the direction my instincts drive me, to such simple visual messages as the flying patterns of birds, I am presented with a vast array of information to decipher. If I take this to my altar and explain what I notice, I am responding to these messages already, announcing to Spirit my awareness and understanding of the messages, or my lack thereof.

A PERSONAL RITUAL FOR SAFETY

I remember my first accident in the city of Ouagadougou. It was very humbling because there was no reason why it happened. The intersection was clearly regulated by traffic light. The light giving me the right of way had turned green a number of seconds before I entered the intersection. I was halfway across when someone on a motorcycle hit me from the side.

In Africa when two people collide in a traffic accident, they usually engage in a fistfight until their tempers cool off before they actually deal with the accident proper. Because I was right, I thought I was entitled to decide whether I wanted a quarrel or not. But the man who hit me did not wait. He postured and gesticulated, then hit me a couple of times while swearing.

I was about to retaliate when he asked point-blank, "Is it your first time in the city?" I said yes. "Did you pay your dues to Mammy Wata?" he continued. I had no idea who Mammy Wata was. Besides, I did not remember anyone telling me to pay anything to anybody, so I said no. The man looked at me and mumbled as if to himself, "No wonder. For there is no way my brand-new brakes would fail me right at this moment." He then departed on his bike after pointing his finger at me and saying I should keep out of his way.

Later on, I learned that the famous Mammy Wata was one of the guardian spirits of the city and that anyone who enters the city for the first time must make a sacrificial give-away to one of the countless people living on the streets before doing anything. This way the travelers are protected because they are in touch with the city vibration. Because I had not done that, I was already in trouble in the Other World, and it was just a matter of time before this trouble would break into this world. Since then, every time I arrive in a new city, I feel obligated to make a give-away.

COMMUNITY RITUALS

Our awareness of a personal connection to the ancestral and spiritual world helps us to build an awareness that prepares us for community ritual. Community ritual can succeed only when every member of the community maintains a personal spiritual connection. Most of the problems I have encountered in community ritual work come from the fact that the people involved had little or no background in doing ritual by themselves. As a result, their attitude and expectations are sometimes quite distant from what is needed for a healing community ritual.

The first thing to recognize is that in community ritual, one is required to give something to the gathering. It takes the combined energies of many givers to make a ritual work. Giving in the context of ritual is the same as participating. All community rituals have certain things in common, such as singing, dancing, and healing. The easiest gift is singing. As they say in indigenous Africa, if you know how to talk, you know how to sing, and if you know how to walk you know how to dance.

The most destructive thing one can do in ritual is to become a passive observer, thinking that your physical presence is enough. In ritual, passivity results in a significant and sometimes dangerous draining of energy. Yet it is frequently seen in community ritual, and it is the issue from which conflict most frequently and predictably arises. When passive participants are reminded that they are not being productive, their usual response is to take offense. It is as if the ego feels the need to protect itself from something it does not know very well. The worst expression of this kind of conflict occurs when people justify their passivity by citing sources they believe to be authoritative about ritual. They quote some expert to prove that being called on to do things one way or another is abusive. Needless to say, people are very creative when it comes to protecting the interests of their ego.

In any community ritual, passivity is the first problem to be aware of because it has countless ways to manifest itself. It forces some people to fold their arms on their chest and stay immobile. Other people act tired and find a seat in a corner, where they wait for everything to end. Still others remain quiet in defiance of what is going on as if saying, "Come get me." It is better to enter into community ritual with people who are familiar with ritual, and with whom you know passivity will not be a problem. In a context of familiarity, there is usually an abundance of generosity. People grab the opportunity to be loving and to be of service to one another inside the ring of a ritual space. They suddenly receive permission from the sacred to love and care for one another in a way not possible in the profane world. This is the closest one can get to village ritual in this culture. But if it is not possible to enter into community ritual with people you know, it is imperative to make the aim of the ritual so strong that it forces people to come together as if they've known one another a long time.

One thing that brings all people together is loss and the fear of loss. When the space shuttle *Challenger* exploded, the entire country came together spontaneously in what amounted to an enormous community ritual. More recently, the death of Princess Diana galvanized people's emotions, so that even people who never expected they would behave this way sat transfixed before the funeral proceedings. The outpouring of emotion at the deaths of all of these figures demonstrated that the most vital cord that links people, even in an individualistic culture, is still emotion. The purpose of the ritual must be sufficiently specific and concrete to draw emotion from its participants. As suggested earlier, people in the West must reconcile with their dead and negotiate with them a serious and lasting peace. The West's constant production of death is a direct manifestation of the denial of it. Reconciliation with the dead, then, is one issue that can motivate people to come together with real emotional intensity.

Another area that binds people together in ritual is personal empowerment and recognition. It is feeling the support of an entire community that provides each person the capacity to pursue his or her gifts and true purpose. When we take a closer look at earth rituals we will see how they can be a place of empowerment. Because earth rituals are a place where people have the opportunity to be seen, appreciated, and loved, earth rituals can facilitate an almost spontaneous coming together. Imagine a group of people coming together to give something to one another in such a way that each person leaves the ritual space feeling confident and reassured. It is an effective way to fuel people's confidence and self-esteem in a manner that allows a much greater involvement of each in the community.

One way to accomplish this is to allow each person the opportunity during the ritual to move to the center of the group in order to receive the group's attention, respect, and appreciation. The responsibility of the group becomes honoring each of its members by articulating her or his special qualities. The members may know they have these qualities, but it becomes apparent in ritual that many of a person's qualities have never been appreciated or even publicly acknowledged. This ritual chases out of the consciousness any self-defeating thought and replaces it with confidence and positive attitude. The choreographic details of how best to accomplish this should be left to the group to decide.

People in the West do not need to form "tribes" in order to do rituals. They simply need to come together with a clear vision. Once together, they will always find a reason to do a ritual, because there is always one problem or another challenging the life of one or many of the group members. Because there is no specific ritual assigned to every single problem, the requirement is the awareness of the power of symbol and symbolic gesture. This means that families, association, workers in the same company can easily develop appropriate rituals for themselves with very little guidance.

PREPARING FOR RITUAL

In summary, learning to conduct ritual means preparing psychologically for ritual—becoming aware of the many challenges one faces when entering a ritual space. These challenges can include the preconceptions and cultural conditioning that we have discussed, such as fear of losing one's identity in the midst of ritual. I have found it useful to suggest that people fight against their own resistance by remembering precisely why they made the choice at the beginning to face a ritual. Rituals break barriers and bring people together in ways they least expect. In ritual it is not difficult and does not take much time for people to come to know one another deeply. That knowledge alone renders unnecessary most coercive forms of community protection, such as a police force and legal system, because, through ritual, Spirit becomes the protective force that preserves the community.

I must reiterate the idea that conducting ritual begins by being acquainted with symbolic objects and gestures. If the psyche cannot be educated to embrace symbolism, people will have difficulty understanding and appreciating rituals. Ritual transcends language and enables us to communicate and interact with the Other World. It is important when conducting ritual that people move out of the literal and dwell as long as possible in the metaphoric and symbolic regions of human experience. This is where the soul and the spirit reside. This is the place where people abandon argument and where superficiality does not intrude. In the world of metaphor and symbol, a simple song and a little rhythm produce far greater results than a panel discussion by articulate experts. Here one experiences true collaboration and learns how to give the attention that all people, all spirits, and all ancestors need.

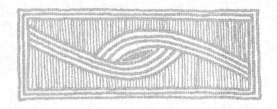

PART FOUR

RITUALS

OF

HEALING

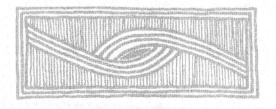

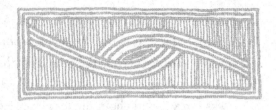

10.

Fire Rituals

Love and sharing will grow in you,
as will the creative fire
to find the means of expressing them.
Fire melts and tempers;
let the fire of love do the same with you.
—Spirit of Fire: To Honor the Earth

The first time I was involved in a fire ritual in the village, I was not told at first that it was a fire ritual. So I thought it was just an exciting nightly gathering with a lot of fire so we could see and talk to one another, since nights in the village are usually very black. My first fire ritual was ecstatic and hot. It took place in the woods outside of the village during a hunting expedition that lasted two nights and three days. As we stopped in a farmland at the end of the day to rest, I noticed that people were gathering dry millet stems and making piles of them. At first I paid no attention to the activity because it is usual to make a bonfire at night when you are sleeping out in order to cook the meat from the game that has been caught during the day. I was not one of the lucky ones who had killed an animal, but I was not worried about dinner because other people were going to share their catch.

What caught my attention was a ring of ash around the pile of millet stems. This meant that something sacred was going to happen. I thought it would be an offering to the nature spirit of one of the animals killed. I had not gone on a long hunting expedition before because I had only recently returned to the village and been initiated as an adult. Finally a cousin of mine, who must have seen my curiosity, told me bluntly that we were going to have a fire ritual. I remembered my experience with the fire at the beginning of initiation, when I felt myself swallowed up by flames and went into an intense dream where I was the only one alive. But my cousin said this one would be different. And indeed it was. This was a ritual of fire shared by villagers of all ages, and its purpose was to keep us connected to the purpose of our expedition, the finding of food for the village. But of course I didn't know all that at the beginning.

Two men my age sat next to the pile of millet stems. One of them produced a pair of fire stones, and the other a piece of cotton. The stones collided against each other and released a spark that fell on the cotton, igniting it. The burning cotton was placed under the pile of stems. Shortly after this I could see a thin filament of white smoke protruding through the dark, then followed by a flame. As the fire grew bigger, hunters gathered around it and began singing an old unfamiliar—to me—village song, and it took me a few minutes to become caught up in it.

The carcass of a bobcat killed during the day was brought to the fire. The hunter who killed it knelt very close to the flame, his eyes wide open and transfixed. He stared at the fire for a long time while we all sang, standing in a circle around the fire. Then he lifted the bobcat high above the flame and let it fall into the flame, which dimmed for a short moment before resuming its brightness. The song accelerated and was met by the smell of burning flesh, which made me hungry. The man who offered his catch of the day to the fire remained in the same posture for a time—long enough for someone to roast. I was concerned for him, but I saw that he was only sweating heavily. At that moment the oldest of the group marched forward and sprinkled the man with water. His body shook briefly and he stood up, bowed to the fire, and walked away from it.

Immediately, another man took his position at the same place. He too had something in his hand. It looked like a piece of meat. The burning millet stems sent a roaring flame that almost licked his bare chest. He stiffened, and his face looked almost convulsed. But he stayed. I noticed that the song grew louder as he struggled with the fire. Surely the melody coming out of twenty-three throats had something to do with his being able to cope with the flames. At last, he threw his piece of meat into the fire. At the same time, the man who carried the water came forward and sprinkled him as he stood up, turned around, and joined the rest of us. I noticed that he did not bow to the fire.

Another man took position. He had nothing in his hands, though his demeanor was the same as the previous two. His eyes locked onto the burning flames for a while, then he stretched his hands toward the flames as if to pray. His lips were moving, though no one could hear what he was saying because everyone was singing. When he received the water and left the space for another person, I noticed his eyes were wet. From then on I watched people take turns at the fire for what felt like a very long time. Some faces that appeared at the fire were familiar, and it was clear that some people were approaching the fire a second time. I decided it was time for me to take a turn, though I did not have enough instruction to understand what I was supposed to do.

As I knelt three feet from the flame, it was hard to believe that anyone could withstand so much heat. My body convulsed as a blanket of heat enveloped it and my mind stopped thinking. I wanted to get out of there, but I felt like I was encased by a wall of melody. The singing worked sometimes like a cooling force, sometimes like a prison that held me tight. Right in front of me was this large river of light with infinite colors. It attracted me, though at the same time I knew I was burning. My worry forced me to pray to the spirit of my grandfather. I asked for protection in this experience, not knowing whether I meant the hunting experience or the fire experience. My eyes were burning with heat, so I shut them. But the sight of the flames was still there, hot and burning. I decided to get up and go, but I could not move. My knees felt as if they were being held from under the ground. I was soaking wet when I came to, and I was sitting on the ground away from the fire and surrounded by a few men. They were still singing, and people were still approaching the fire. I noticed that some people were eating while others were singing. The ritual had turned festive with the inclusion of food. Soon everybody joined in the dinner around the very fire that had cooked us all. My cousin warned me that next time I should not try to stay so long next to the open fire.

I came away from this ritual feeling lighter and very energized. I knew I had stayed there long enough to have burns, but I had none. So I became aware that the fire had burned something else in me instead of my flesh. The idea that fire does not have to burn hit my mind, and I became aware that I can choose what I want fire to consume inside of me. I also realized that this is the kind of functional fire I needed in my life—the fire that burns away all undesirable things that get attached to me in my life journey. Their periodic incineration at the fire ritual allows me to feel less weighted down.

We begin with rituals of fire, because fire is the first element in the Dagara cosmic wheel. Fire is the element that keeps people connected to their purpose and to the world of Spirit. However, it is extremely dangerous to suggest a fire ritual to people in the West, because Western society's essential characteristic is fire, and Westerners therefore need to understand the power of fire more than they need to perform rituals of fire. Positive fire, as we saw in the earlier chapter, emerges as vision, dream, and intimacy with the ancestors. Negative fire is speed, restlessness, radical consumption, and eventually death. Because the attributes of fire in the West are predominantly negative, people need to attend to that which can stabilize their fire before they move on to exploring fire as the warmth of

being, creativity, and life. Therefore, before most Westerners interest
themselves in fire rituals, it is crucial that they make their peace with water. (The next chapter focuses on a variety of water rituals that work well
in the modern world.) I include one fire ritual here, so that readers may
glimpse the healing potential of such a ritual, but more important for
Westerners than undertaking such a ritual is understanding the purposes
of fire and the consequences of letting its negative attributes rage out of
control.

ATTRIBUTES OF FIRE

In the indigenous mind, fire kindles and sustains an animating and pervasive energy in all that lives. It is in the water that runs, it is in the trees, the
rocks, the earth, and in ourselves. It is the mediator between worlds since
it is very close to the purest form of energy. Any connection with ancestors, spirits and the Other World is mediated by fire. A complete understanding of fire requires a serious relationship with death, and the dead.
Because fire burns, those who relate to fire are often tense and must be
clear about their intention in working with the fire. The tension referred
to here is like a charge of energy about to burst. Those who carry such
fiery energy are being prepared for energetic action that reflects, and is the
result of, a touch from the Other World.

Fire is the rising force that makes us do, see, feel, love, and hate. Fire
has great power, both outside of us and within us. On the outside, visible
fire drives us to perform our respective duties, to fulfill our life purpose.

But a fire burns also within us. The fire within connects us to our real
family—the people we are always drawn to when we see them—and
causes them to recognize us. This fire originates in the Other World and
connects us always to the ancestors. Through the fire within we can converse with those we left behind in the Other World by being born here.
The inner fire is a rope that connects us to the world we abandoned when
we were born into a human body. To the indigenous, that world is our real

home. This does not mean that this world is not real. It is a place we pass through.

The way to move to a productive understanding of and relationship with fire is through ritual, where fire is experienced not as a combustive fire, but as a warm, comforting, and loving fire connecting us to the ancestors in the Other World. At the core of the fire ritual is the indigenous belief that each person is born with a purpose, and that this purpose was presented to the council of the ancestors in the Spirit World for approval prior to each person's journey to Earth. We come into the world in order to bring to completion that very plan which, as we are born into this side of reality, became our reason for human life. In order to fulfill our purpose, we need the driving force of fire, just as a vehicle needs fuel to reach its destination.

Two things here are at work. We must remember what we came here to do, and we must have a community that knows and remembers our purpose and supports it fully. We do not want a community that tells us what it thinks we should do, but a community that unconditionally provides for us in a manner that allows us to accept our responsibilities and realize the life of our purpose.

From an indigenous point of view, every time a situation pushes us to move faster than is appropriate, every time our heart beats more quickly than normal, every time we get excited for one reason or another, we become situated in the fiery origin, that chaotic place at the time of the beginning of the world. To be ill is therefore to be en route toward that origin; it implies heat, activity, friction, and struggle. It also calls attention to the fact that the encounter between fire and water that resulted in the creation of our earth and life is not to be taken for granted. The kind of balance required for the maintenance of peace and reconciliation is so tenuous that we are constantly thrown back toward tense and chaotic fiery states. Many circumstances of our lives can send us toward the chaotic fire, such as death, accident, shocks to our life that we connect with. It is the indigenous understanding that we attract these circumstances in order to push us forward to a deeper transformation. The indigenous does not believe in coincidences or in accidents.

WHEN FIRE IS MISALIGNED

The power of fire must be aimed toward something through focused intention, or fire becomes misaligned in the psyche and in society. For example, a person who constantly attracts or makes trouble has his or her fire misaligned. Correction of the person's behavior would have to be ritualistic, that is, it would take place in a ritual similar to the one outlined above. When the tension produced by fire is not focused, it produces an extreme and often destructive tension in the world. When the fire within a person produces only fire in the world around them, the result is most often violence and death.

The fiery temperament of the world and particularly the West has resulted in a great deal of spilling of blood, both symbolic and literal. Indigenous people see the death that results from war or accident as sacrifices to fire, just as the animal killed in the hunt was offered to the fire as a sacrifice. But the engine of fire in the West appears, to indigenous people, to be the technological machine, which consumes nature around the world. Villagers see the fire of technology consuming both through its speed (as in accidental deaths of animals near highways) and through the capitalist accumulation of land and rape of natural resources.

From an indigenous point of view, Westerners are sacrificing much to fires that rage out of control. Just as fire consumes everything in its path, so consumers in the West sacrifice the life of Spirit for an endless pursuit of material goods. Material consumption does not provide care for the soul. It is as if misaligned inner fire is encouraged and supported in modern culture, something necessary to boost production and consumption. When adequately programmed through advertising and the media, people want to accumulate items because such items are regarded as an opportunity for fulfillment. Driven by an internal fire that cannot be quenched, the modern consumer is like a greyhound racing for fulfillment. The goal becomes not so much to reach a destination as to stay in your lane and keep running. When this inner fire is not connected to its source, it drives people to race endlessly after things that do not matter.

For this reason—the fact that fire can become so easily misaligned—I have hesitated before outlining for Westerners how to do fire rituals. From the point of view of my people, the growth, expansion, and progress by which the modern world measures success is a conflagration, a fire burning out of control and consuming everything it touches. It is essential that the modern world stop burning itself and the rest of the planet, and to learn to see beyond the notion of fire that can only consume, to see the aspects of fire that can lead to transformation, healing, and a renewed connection to the world of the ancestors and Spirit that holds our purpose.

To begin making their peace with fire, Westerners must notice the common symptoms of fire in their milieu. In the modern world, being out of alignment with fire translates into pollution of one sort or another. It is as if to be civilized, one must infect the air, leak oil into the waters, and seek to move faster today than we did yesterday. Once we understand this as symptomatic of a state of disconnection, then it becomes possible to seek reconnection and reconciliation with the past. Changing our intention from consumption, as an out-of-control fire, to connection, like a fire that warms and soothes, will bring fire in Western culture under control to a very great extent.

It is reconciling oneself with the past—or, as the Dagara would say, with the ancestors—that brings the inner fire into alignment. The work of grieving is an important part of reconciling with the past, and for that reason I suggest that water rituals precede fire rituals in the West. The work of building relationships in community also contributes to the taming of fire, for in order to have healthy relationships, one must have made peace with the past. One must also tame the inner fire simply in order to live in community, for close relationships breed a friction that would rage out of control if the friends or partners had not done a great deal of work with their psyches.

When an individual is not in alignment with fire, there is chaos and contradiction in that person's behavior patterns. There is a tendency to be fearful of fire, yet there is an almost irresistible attraction to fire. This confusion comes from a lack of harmony between the fires that burn within the person and the way that this fiery energy is expressed and manifested in the outer world. A fire ritual can allow us to experience the positive energies of fire without this chaos and fear.

In a fire ritual, one takes a good look at the intensity of the Other World. In the world of magic, heat opens doors. I remember times in the course of initiation rituals when the heat alone would rise to the point where it would open a window into the Other World, and one would glimpse spirit beings. At those times I was able to see, and also to understand, what tribal wisdom means when it declares that divine or ancestral heat comes to us from below, not from above. It was easy to see why god cannot be above the clouds; god is here underneath our feet. The opening was of the earth, not of the sky. The faces that appeared in the heat were ancestral faces peeking into this world.

The heat of the fire ritual also reminds us that heat is the circulation of energy. Life is manifested only when energy can circulate. The Dagara language uses the same word *di* (prounounced "dee") to mean "burn," "consume," and "eat." The connection is not, however, about destruction, but about transformation. Any person who goes through a fire ritual involves himself with transformation and change.

An example of a healing fire ritual follows.

A FIRE RITUAL

In a fire ritual, the fire must be looked at as a bond to the world of the ancestors and spirits, not just as a bonfire, because its function is to put people on track, not to burn them off track. The content of the ritual itself must be twofold. First is the casting into the fire of that which is known to interfere with our focus. In other words, the burning fire must consume that which stands between us and the purpose that determines the course of our lives. Next we must reiterate our commitment to walking our life's path by taking time to commune with the fire, asking that it transform that which it has just consumed into whatever it is we need to thrive and grow and continue.

The great power of fire can be very frightening, and during a ritual the intensity of its heat can feel threatening, but fire is what is needed by those who have lost connection to their purpose. The fire ritual aims at responding to someone who is extremely creative, has a lot of ideas and projects, but who is mysteriously blocked from being able to carry them out. Here in the West, this might take the form of someone who is always frantically busy, while running away from things they don't want to see in their life.

So let us take a small group of about ten people interested in a fire ritual. Each has prepared ahead of time a symbol of what needs to be released into the fire and has brought this object, which the fire can burn. It could simply be a piece of paper containing the written version of what needs to be thrown away, or a symbolic item of almost any flammable form.

It is preferable that the ritual happen at night, for when it is dark the full meaning of fire is revealed. The group will begin by building a fireplace, which will be their shrine. One of them must be selected as a fire keeper. He or she will be the person in charge of maintaining the fire at its proper intensity during the ritual. Another person, the ritual leader or facilitator, will be in charge of the general choreography or proceedings.

With the group standing, gathered in any formation around the fire to form a bond, the ritual leader leads them in an invocation. In the invocation, the purpose of the ritual must be clearly stressed and stated. Names of allies in the world of Spirit must be called. More specifically, ancestors known and unknown must be invited to take part in the effort to reconnect with the purposes that burn within. The ritual leader would initiate this, then allow for each participant to invite in those personal helping spirits and ancestors that they wish to be present to assist with the ritual. Next, each participant would be urged to communicate to the group the obstacle he or she intends to overcome. Putting the problem into words destabilizes it and loosens its grip on the psyche, making it possible to give it over to the fire for transformation.

At the completion of the invocation, each participant, one at a time, must move close to the fire and experience the heat while keeping their attention focused on the blaze, very conscious of what must be released into the fire. The object that each brought is surrendered to the fire. It is now the time to come to full grips with one's life commitment by devoting undivided attention to the burning fire and embracing the heat.

The time each person spends in close proximity to the fire is determined by their need. It is preferable that while there, the rest of the group be engaged in some common activity such as chanting and drumming. Every time an individual completes his or her time before the fire, he is warmly welcomed back into the group with gentle touch and embraces. The assumption here is that each person will return to the group in an emotional state. Such a person needs to experience acceptance. So as each person completes his part and becomes, as a result, a transformed person, it is the responsibility of the rest of the group to demonstrate its ability to give love, attention, and caring to them. This completes the reintegration of the person. Without this, the person is left feeling very much alone, wondering why they ever submitted to the risk of ritual.

After each person has approached the fire and returned to the others, the group moves closer to the flame as a single entity, and closes the ritual with a word of gratitude to the ancestors and spiritual allies present at the occasion. The fire ceremony is over.

It is useful at the end of the fire ritual to introduce water, for the heat of tension and intention must be monitored and constrained by water so that the fire may transform and not simply incinerate. If, for example, the fire ritual is done near the shore of a stream or lake, immersion of everyone in water afterward is a good idea.

A fire ritual is a place where things that interfere with our connection with our soul's purpose can be surrendered, and where fire can serve as a point of focus. The result of this ritual is usually a sense of orientation and even calmness symptomatic of a certain level of harmony with Spirit. An outer fire in the sacred space of a ritual has the power to stop an inner fire from consuming everything by producing a moderating force that counters the appetite for speed and restlessness. When this happens, people wake up from their stupor and become able to distinguish between pursuits that fulfill their purpose and pursuits that do not.

Fire must be redefined to become an instrument that offers the possibility of connection, and fire rituals must be seen within this context, where they help renew and strengthen one's relationship with the past, present and future. One cannot maintain this focus without discovering in it the active role of the ancestors in one's life and becoming as clear as possible about their own purpose. This is why I think a catalog of fire rituals for people to choose from is not as important as a deep understanding of the fire that blazes within, and of how, when neglected, this fire drives the modern world to destruction in the interest of progress.

To moderate the effects of fire, modern people need rituals of water, and to these we now turn.

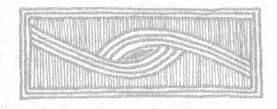

11.

Water Rituals

Last night, as I was sleeping,
I dreamt—marvelous error!—
that a spring was breaking
out in my heart.
I said: Along which secret aqueduct,
Oh water, are you coming to me,
water of a new life
that I have never drunk?
—ANTONIO MACHADO, "Last Night,"
translated by Robert Bly

Water rituals focus on water's cosmological and symbolic meaning. Doing a water ritual means that one sees water as representing more than the sum of its chemical components. The amount of water and how it is used determine the nature and power of the ritual. For example, a libation is simply the pouring out of a small quantity of water to anyone in the Spirit World for the purpose of encouraging peace and togetherness. This seemingly simple act indicates that one wishes to make peace, to be in harmony with someone or something else. A libation is a maintenance ritual that can be done at any time.

On the other hand, full immersion in water, especially cold water, is considered a radical ritual aimed at producing massive cathartic results. The recipient of this catharsis experiences a new beginning. Either way, water ritual is an attempt to unite things that must be united, to reconcile things that are meant to be together in the interest of community. Water rituals tie up loose ends. These loose ends are obstacles to our balance and reconciliation, our peace and serenity.

WATER RITUALS AND HEALING

We have described water as the second element in the cosmological wheel, a key element that at the beginning cooled the raging fires and brought stability, reorienting the cosmic energy toward producing continuity and community. Since then, people all over the world have felt the need to return again and again to water for purification, cleansing, reconciling, and making peace in the face of the onslaught of life's challenges.

This means that to the indigenous, challenge or crisis is cosmologically and spiritually symptomatic of a rise in fire. When someone is in crisis, regardless of the nature of the crisis, that person is said to be returning to fire. The distress of the person drifting toward or into fire is a plea for the radically reconciling introduction of water. When there is no water around, we are vulnerable to crisis. People, especially people in crisis, are naturally attracted to water. Many recognize that when they are agitated about something in their lives, they find peace at the waterfront. Just the sight of a large body of water brings a feeling of quiet and peace, a feeling of home. Water resets a system gone dry in which motion is accelerated beyond what we can bear. African healing wisdom looks at physical illness as a fire moving a person's energy beyond the limit of what he or she can bear. This suggests that we all need water, and need rituals of water, to stay balanced, oriented, and reconciled.

There are countless aspects of human experience that water rituals affect in a healing way. One of them, perhaps the most important, is the emotional self. Many people in the Western world walk around like time bombs, loaded with contradictory emotions that are often so hard to articulate that the individual is dangerous to himself and to his surroundings. Perhaps first among these emotions is grief. In this culture, the challenge of confronting overwhelming grief must be considered the most crucial task requiring the reconciling energy of water.

In indigenous Africa, one cannot conceive of a community that does not grieve. In my village, people cry every day. Until grief is restored in the West as the starting place where the modern man and woman might find peace, the culture will continue to abuse and ignore the power of water, and in turn will be fascinated with fire. Grief must be approached as a release of the tension created by separation and disconnection from someone or something that matters. The average Western person is grieving about being isolated. Western men in particular are grieving about the dead they didn't grieve properly because they were told that men don't cry. In my work, I hear this everywhere. Grief is not only expressed in tears, but also in anger, rage, frustration, and sadness. An angry person is a person on the road to tears, the softer version of grief. Sadness and the feeling of heaviness within are symptomatic of a deep well of grief in the psychic underground.

One must ask why tears, the softest expression of grief, are not as acceptable in the modern world as are anger and rage. I say this because to indigenous Africans emotions are sacred. To villagers it looks as if the West is uncomfortable with tears because one cannot argue verbally, logically, against this kind of emotion. Villagers also believe that Westerners are afraid of emotion because they are afraid of loss of control. Emotions have the tendency to spread from person to person, and therefore social control, to the Western mind, is being risked with any display of emotion.

Many Westerners are beginning to see that there is also danger in remaining stuck with rage, anger, and sadness; they are the directionless vehicles of a grief that remains hidden. When these emotions are not allowed a fluid catharsis, one is left in a state of incompleteness. The end of the domination of one's life by such emotions requires an outpouring of liquid. You cannot truly grieve within and remain composed without. Emotion is an extroverted phenomenon, and it cannot find its much-needed release if expressed only internally. Denied an outward expression, grief grows stronger and organizes itself like a hurricane that can rise up and sweep us away. I have heard many times people express their fear of grief because they feel that if they even begin to release it, they will be overcome, eventually drowning in their own tears. Indeed, this is how it feels, but this is not what actually happens.

In my village, emotion is ritualized because it is seen as a sacred thing. If addressed within a sacred space, the emotions of grief can provide powerful relief and healing. Any time the feeling of loss arises, there is an energy that demands ritual in order to allow reconciliation and the return of peace. These are crises that water rituals can resolve. Water rituals help to shed the massive accumulation of negative emotion due to loss, failure, and powerlessness. Each one of these problems heightens our awareness of the challenges of life. Loss and powerlessness are particularly humbling because they disrupt continuity and reveal our humanity. One of the things all humans have in common is loss, be it the loss of loved ones or the loss of dreams, be it the loss of a job or a relationship. In all of these situations, water rituals are necessary.

In order to do a water ritual effectively, one needs a community. There are few personal water rituals, as the Dagara people don't comprehend the idea of private grief. Grief is a community problem because the person who is sick belongs to the entire community. Just as a wound on your leg cannot be approached as the leg's problem alone, but must be treated as a problem for the entire body, a person in a village who is sick with grief sickens the rest of the village.

A COMMUNAL GRIEF RITUAL

Let us then go to a ritual involving someone who is struggling with some serious loss such as one of those named above. The central water element here is tears, because we are talking about loss. The group would come together around that person, forming a village to help him or her heal from the loss by going together into the person's grief. The responsibility of this village is to show the person that her or his loss is a loss for the entire village.

The success of the water ritual is ensured by the presence of intense, focused attention. It is therefore the group's responsibility to know as much about the person as possible. The village gathers in a circle, placing the person in the middle. At the core of the ritual is the person communicating to the village the story of his or her loss. The person's story of loss triggers a variety of spoken responses from the villagers, with each response reemphasizing the story told by the person. Attention and emphasis in the responses must be on why this loss has chosen to befall this person and what is it saying to all of us. I have to reiterate that the indigenous address events, illness, natural disasters as if they are living entities. So a person with a fever could talk to the fever. And in the case of loss, the person in the center of the ritual says something to the effect that his or her house burned down, stirring up the feeling of homelessness. The response from one person will come in the form of a question directed at Spirit and emphasizing the emotional wound caused to a brother or a sister in this sad event. Another one will confirm that the burning still continues and is in fact burning everyone into exile. One after another, people will expand this symbol, stretching the loss of the one into the loss of the many. After deploring the loss and the paralysis that it produces, the villagers must each speak about something in the person that is irreplaceable to the community. One after another, the villagers tell the person about how the village cannot survive or continue without him or her. This statement must be substantiated with examples from the person's life. Every statement is punctuated with spontaneous collective grieving.

The philosophy behind this is that visibility and recognition are sources of empowerment, while anonymity leads to self-doubt and eventually to failure. People need to hear good things about themselves told to them with sincerity, honesty, and integrity. There is a force in this that allows the person to thrive. There is nothing like being seen within this kind of light. The healing comes when the sick energy that grows in the darkness of isolation becomes upset by such intense recognition. After a little struggle and resistance, it rushes away, leaving its victim feeling liberated. In almost every case, many tears are involved.

In a ritual involving a much larger crowd, there is no time or adequate structure to provide individualized attention. Instead of a circle, people gather as a throng in an egg-shaped space, one end of which is designated as the village, and the other end as the shrine. The egg form befits a water ritual because it represents life in formation. It symbolizes the process of creating order. The village area is the place of gathering emotion. There, people focus the energy of their emotion. The shrine is the where the highly charged emotion must be released.

The shrine must be built carefully. Usually a community shrine will have a stature proportional to the size of the community. For instance you would not produce a miniature water ritual shrine for a village of a hundred or more people. The average village is about 150 people. This means that a shrine would normally have the size of a hut. And indeed, the shrine can look like a hut cut in half vertically. It is built using elements freshly borrowed from Mother Nature, such as tree branches, plants, flowers, and so forth. Its form depends on the creativity of the village, but more often than not, a shrine of this sort will look like a gateway with an arched form atop a wide base. The surface of the base serves as the doorway to the Other World, and as such it requires the reverence and respect due such a gateway. Here in the West, the shrine would be best if it reflects the imagination of the people who are building it. This is not prescriptive but rather suggestive.

The egg-shaped space between the village and the shrine is arranged as a place of chaos. By this I mean that there is no organized path for the human traffic. Here people loaded with emotion will walk toward the shrine, intending to unload the weight of grief into the Other World. Others walk back to the village after relieving themselves of their burden at the shrine. There is no prescribed way of unloading emotion, just as one cannot dictate how emotion is expressed. People should feel free to follow their instinct in this matter. The overall sense is of a volume of moving human traffic. The middle space, filled with the back-and-forth motion of people, symbolizes possibilities, the possibility of access between one world and another. It is also a linking agent, a conduit and place of hope.

Once the ritual space has been prepared along these lines, the villagers begin their inner preparation. It is sometimes useful for them to get together in small groups of eight to twelve people to tell one another what causes them grief. This is because grief does not necessarily come on demand. It is something that must be evoked through stories and images. One of the ways of triggering emotion is to speak about it or to hear it spoken about by others. Before telling the stories of grief, each small group first makes a prayer to Spirit, requesting its presence to help pluck out that which causes tension, paralysis, and distress. The purpose is to help break the seal of grief, creating the atmosphere conducive to emotion. Each person should have brought an object symbolic of his or her loss, which will be described in the form of a story to the rest of the group. Usually deep emotions are shared in the course of these preparations even before the general gathering. Every grief story has similar elements. This is why one story invites another. This process can take hours.

After everyone has shared their story with their small group, the small groups rejoin to engage in the ritual proper. A strong feeling of emotional tension has already been built, propelling the grieving process forward. Organizing a procession (if space permits) toward the ritual village (the space already prepared for the ritual itself) will symbolize this forward movement. It will also emphasize the depth of the internal journey required in order to heal. A procession also affords an opportunity to experience a kind of pilgrimage, which encourages the flow of emotions even before the cleansing transformation produced by the ritual itself. The human psyche adores the procession and succumbs more easily and naturally to anything that follows. In the mind of the indigenous, human beings are on a journey, a pilgrimage toward the spiritual landscape of enlightenment. Therefore every time there is an opportunity to march, carrying some symbolic objects such as banners, statues, arches, or candles, the spirit is reminded of the connection between the current procession or march and the inner journey that is constantly happening.

The arch usually symbolizes a covenant, some sort of agreement with a higher reality. It could simply be the agreement to heal, or it could represent an affirmation of a people's will to survive onslaughts. Among the Dagara, this arch is usually made in the form of a pyramid and is always symbolic of a covenant with the ancestors. The candle is an opportunity to hold on to one's focus and symbolizes an affirmation of light over darkness. Proceeding toward the symbolic village space helps people unload unwanted emotional residues and serves to deepen alertness to any inner turbulence that may hinder the commitment to heal. This unloading is made possible because the people in it feel the freedom within the ritual setting to let go of any reservations to really experiencing their grief. They might find, for instance, that if they just experienced a severe grief, like a death in the family, that they closed themselves down at some point to expressing their grief openly. Now, during the procession, is the time to reopen themselves, to discover the communal safety that will allow them to continue their process of grieving openly.

When the procession has reached the ritual space, each small group as a unit enters the village. (I use village, ritual village, and symbolic village to mean the same thing.) Once the groups have entered the village, the processional arch is lowered to the ground to reflect the sacredness of the earth upon which the reconciliation takes place. Following this, there must be a prayer to the ancestors, requesting their presence at the ritual, their stamp of approval, and their sanction of its sacredness. Then a rhythmic song of grief must be intoned by someone and taken up by the entire village. The song must be supported by drums. Rhythm and chant are two sustaining ingredients in community rituals. Together they constitute the umbrella overarching the community engaged in this healing journey.

Shortly after engaging in the song, each group must go, one at a time, to the shrine, and each member, one after another, steps forward to place his or her object of grief on the shrine. The shrine is guarded by gatekeepers posted on either side. The actual ritual does not proceed until all the groups have checked in at the shrine, released their bundles, and returned to the village area. The bundles, because they represent the sum total of the losses of the village, together constitute a magnetic point that pulls the emotional self toward it, the same way a light in the dark attracts insects.

Once everyone has gathered in the village, the actual grieving begins. As emotion builds up in people, they move to the shrine and release it, then return to the village to build up again. Any person who, moved by emotion, begins to head toward the shrine must be discreetly accompanied by someone who is not emotionally loaded in order to protect them. There is a danger that a highly emotionally charged person may not distinguish between unloading their emotion and throwing themselves bodily into the shrine. The pull to throw oneself into the shrine is so intense that someone must be there to ensure that only the emotion stays at the shrine and the person returns to the village where she or he belongs. Much praying, lamenting, and grieving takes place. People may spontaneously throw themselves to the ground, convulsing in grief. The danger for a person who has never grieved is that once he or she begins, there is an avalanche of emotion that wants to come out all at once.

It is not recommended to wait in the village until you become like an overinflated balloon of grief before going to the shrine. If you do, you might simply want to end your life by walking into the Other World. Your fascination will be overstimulated by the intensity you carry within. The way one proceeds to the shrine is determined by the intensity of one's feeling. You cannot walk slowly and majestically toward the shrine when you feel as though you are going to explode at any moment. If you are bursting inside, you should rush your burden to the shrine. Similarly, you don't rush an emotion that is not rushing you.

It is the job of the assistant who accompanies the person grieving to look after that person and ensure their safety. The assistant pays attention to the pace she or he is moving, keeping the one grieving from throwing themselves headlong into the gateway to the Other World. The assistant's attention must be demonstrated by his or her ability to maintain the appropriate pace of things.

In the village itself, people, both grievers and nongrievers, sing in unison. Some dance as they feel moved to, and everybody must allow their body to swing to the melody of the chant and to the beat of the drum. Responding to music and rhythm allows emotion to build so that it can be unloaded at the shrine. It is not permitted to cultivate solemnity in the village, because solemnity encourages withdrawal and suspends participation. The village is a place where energy must flow, and stillness opposes that flow. Solemnity encourages stillness and must therefore be discouraged.

There is no telling how long the period of commuting between the village and the shrine will last. As long as there are emotions to be unloaded, the ritual must continue. This is why in Dagara tradition, such a ritual usually takes three days. Meanwhile, other life functions are either suspended or operate at a minimal capacity. When the emotional stream is unleashed, it has to drip itself to dryness before it is stopped. Otherwise one can become sick from repressing emotion. The ritual does not end until it feels as if the emotional force is dissipating. At that time the entire village chants its way to the shrine and continues to chant while a special task force collects all the bundles from the shrine. Each person in this group must be cleansed in some way prior to the collection of bundles. The cleansing is usually done with scented smoke from sage and herbs. While the collection is taking place, smoke is spread as a thick wall between the village and the shrine where the bundles are being gathered.

When the task force finishes collecting the bundles, they walk away with them in a tight formation to a place where they will carefully bury them in the ground. Then they wash themselves someplace where there is natural cold water. Meanwhile the village brings the song to an end and disperses. The villagers will return shortly, usually the next morning, to undo the shrine and return every piece of it to nature. The indigenous believe that only nature can take these pieces and process the energy from them, like a spiritual form of composting.

This type of ritual befits a large group and handles a variety of emotions without attention to too many specific details and without making the individual feel lost and ineffectual. What people share in common is the sense of loss, and this alone is enough to spur them on. A periodic return to this kind of ritual has positive consequences far beyond what words can express. Water is the focus of this type of ritual because it represents reconciliation and the return of balance. In tribal life one does not have to save one's grief, patiently waiting for someone to die. The tribe is big enough to experience death almost on a daily basis, so emotions are released and one is reconciled to loss continually. Villagers gauge the amount of grief that is built up in them by the barometer of their joy. When emotion has been fully unloaded, the rush of joy that fills you up can last for days or weeks. When that feeling of joy subsides, grief is again building and will soon require another release.

A RITUAL OF RECONCILIATION

Another example of a water ritual that has been practiced in a variety of indigenous cultures throughout the African continent is called the reconciliation ritual. This ritual has to do with cleansing and purifying the psyche.

Every year, the village gathers for its reconciliation ritual at the local river. In the water, healers await each villager who comes for healing. As the villager approaches the water, he or she is received by the healers and reminded of the spiritual depth of the event. The villager then enters the water and walks to the main healer, who asks a series of questions about the act of cleansing to ensure that the person seeking healing understands the meaning of cleansing, admits to being in need of it, and acknowledges that it can only be granted by the ancestors. Sometimes a question as blunt as "Do you understand what you're here to do?" is asked to make sure that the person is sincere and is not involved in performing.

The healer then declares to the villager that he or she is not the one who is going to do the healing; this is done by the very spirit that dwells in the water. After this short dialogue, the villager is dunked into the water and kept underwater for as long as they can hold their breath, sometimes a little bit beyond this point to ensure a breakthrough. At this point, the villager is released and dashes out of the water like a bullet, full of emotion. They are then held gently by some assistants and guided back to the village, which welcomes them with a loud cheer. They are a new person. Notice here that the healer does not heal but is like an assistant to the water spirit, who actually does the healing. Indeed, the indigenous believe that real cleansing takes place underwater. The water spirit does not come to you until that moment when you feel very uncomfortable. This is an extension of the belief that every time the Other World is present, everybody should feel uncomfortable.

Missionaries who witnessed these rituals either regarded them as a strange prebiblical paganism or decided that indigenous people were Christians at heart, in need of the blessing of divine guidance. However, to the Dagara, a ritual such as this signifies renewal, rebirth, and purification. The cleansing of a water ritual is seen by indigenous people as something to be done with regularity because of human vulnerability to contamination by negative energy. I do this quite frequently right here in the West.

A RITUAL OF PROSPERITY

The spirit of water is the spirit that watches over the fetus as it develops, promising it a home and the prosperity it needs to fulfill its purpose after it is born. One of the qualities held by the element water is that of focus, and an appeal can be made to water to bring us the focus needed to live the purposeful life that we were born to and to ensure the prosperity sufficient to survive and thrive while living in this purpose. There is a ritual done each year by some villages that could be easily adopted in the West.

A group of people seeking the prosperity that the focus found in water can bring would build a small boat. Decorating the boat becomes a group project, with each person offering something of personal value to the decoration, so that the boat becomes something of great beauty. In the invocation, each person would state what they needed in order to prosper in the coming year, thanking the mother of water for the focus and attention that she brings, and humbly offering their contribution on the boat as a token of their gratitude. The requests should be quite specific and clear, not just a general request for prosperity. At the end of the invocation, with singing, drumming, and general joy the boat is set into a river of running water that runs to the sea.

A RITUAL OF LIBATION

Beside these examples of community water rituals, there is a more private ritual that can be done by anyone needing the continued blessings of peace and good fortune. I referred to it at the beginning of this chapter as a libation. Any water poured to the ancestors or spirit beings is received in the Other World for the purpose of providing peaceful continuity. This is something that can be done as a thank-you to spirits for something they've helped accomplish or for their continued protection.

If you have established a sacred altar in your house, it is recommended that you go there every morning with a glass of fresh cold water. As you sit or kneel at the altar, holding the water in your hand, pray to the spirit of the ancestors and to any spirit being you know, inviting them to be the main artisans of the day ahead of you. It is useful to tell in as much detail as possible what the content of the day is going to be, including meetings that are very important to you, and even express such things as your concerns about commuting in traffic. The focus here is on the activities that you want to be monitored by Spirit. At the end, pour a little water on the altar, asking the ancestors to take it and use it as a peaceful umbrella that protects against the heat of misfortune, bad luck, and disappointment. Leave the glass or a bowl of water on the altar at all times, as the presence of water anywhere indicates your desire for peace, reconciliation, and focus in that place. A day that begins this way offers more happy surprises than bad ones. A libation is salutary every time you face something with a little challenge in it.

A final and even simpler ritual involves simply maintaining a bowl of water someplace where you spend time, such as on an altar, in the house, or at an office. Placing a bowl of water in a room where a difficult discussion or meeting is to take place can have a remarkable effect on the tone of the interaction. The mere presence of water near us is calming and reminds us of the peace and reconciliation we desire in all aspects of our lives.

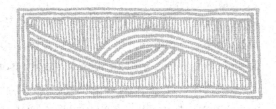

12.

Earth Rituals

Come, listen to the earth with us.
For those who have learned to hear its song
the earth can soothe the troubled heart,
refresh the weary,
soften the hardened,
redirect the lost.
—STEVE VAN MATRE, *The Earth Speaks*

Earth is where we belong. She is our home. She gives us sustenance unconditionally and makes it possible for us to feel connected. Earth is where we go to and where we depart from. This means that she sees us in a way no one can. The nourishment and support of the Earth Mother grant us the feeling of belonging that allows us to expand and grow because we feel strong. Our well-being depends on this feeling of belonging, and perhaps this is why each of us fosters some type of territorial instinct, wishing to protect that which nourishes us. Earth's protection reflects her undivided commitment to us. We, in turn, protect her because she defines us and provides us with an abundance of resources.

Earth rituals greatly emphasize the sense of belonging, self-worth, and community, including all forms of relationships. They serve as an opportunity for a group of people to demonstrate their ability to give attention, love, appreciation, and caring to an individual who needs it badly. This is how certain psychological illnesses are healed. Our womb is the earth; it is our place of origination. Feelings of absence, of being out of touch, any form of alienation, anonymity, and purposelessness—all are symptomatic of a disconnection with the earth. No other element can heal the hollow psyche in search of fulfillment, and for such situations, earth rituals are required.

EARTH RITUALS AND TOUCH

One aspect of earth ritual that people in the West are clearly in need of involves touching. Human hands carry a huge amount of healing energy, provided that one is aware of the kind of mental alignment that must accompany their touch. Our hands are healing instruments that must be treated as sacred. Many modern psychological and physical illnesses are linked to energetic depletion due to "touchless" surroundings. When the individualism of the West results in physical and emotional isolation from others, as it often does, people can become so starved for touch that their need can translate into severe physical illness. Isolated from others, people become afraid of touch, especially unsolicited touch. But a person's level of concern about being touched is almost always proportional to his or her need for it.

There is a deeply sacred dimension to touch, and therefore, a ritual that authorizes people to touch one another allows them to relax in a sacred context. So there is a need to reacquaint people with the sacredness of touch. In my village, for instance, children spend their early years on the backs of their mothers or baby-sitters. Wherever they go, they hang on their back comfortably, enjoying the warm protection of their guardian's body. At night they sleep in the same bed with their parents. This continuous availability of touch nourishes something in the person's psyche that is fundamental to a future sense of community. The person later becomes aware of what a sense of belonging is and can't think of himself or herself outside of a community with other people.

I believe strongly that people who crave community in this country also crave the healing touch of human hands. The road to a real sense of community begins with the ability to restore the amount of touch that the body has been denied since the beginning of its human journey. The craving of the body for what is vaguely known as love corresponds to the need for filling up the great hole left in the psyche by a lack of tender physical contact. Restoring touch will help make it possible to stay in touch.

When people get together, the initial enjoyment of the encounter comes from their psyches touching one another energetically at close proximity. I have noticed among Westerners, however, that the intensity of the need for connection with another person competes with a powerful ambivalence about touch that often leads to an exasperating shallowness of communication and interaction. One sees this quite literally between two people who love each other but who are in conflict. They fail to recognize that their difficulties may have nothing to do with one of them being wrong about issues between them. What they are really troubled by is the lack of being touched.

The lack of touch is the greatest source of grief in modern culture. Poor self-esteem and the shrinking of a person's sense of identity can be traced, in part, to the lack of touch. But the restoration of touch must be done properly and not as a way of trying to stop a person from experiencing any emotion he or she needs to experience in the interest of healing. It also must avoid becoming a vulture's gesture, intended to consume an outpouring of energy. The danger is that when touch does not actually give energy to another person, it absorbs it, or scares it into protective silence. The person guilty of such energetic felonies may not even be aware of what they are doing.

In a context in which deprivation from touch is the rule, people grieve and crave secretly. This internal grieving is dangerous because it attacks the psyche and breeds more negative energy within. The opportunity to cry can trigger a healing process that touch accelerates if it is offered wisely and thoughtfully. The hungriest person inside us is not the one who is thinking about dinner, but the one who has not felt loved for a long time. This is why in Africa, amid scarcity of the worst sort, people still manage to wear a smile, to be genuinely generous and hospitable. While their physical stomachs are empty, their psychic bellies are overfilled with the food of touch.

It is not possible to engage in a productive earth ritual without proper touch. Earth is the archetypal symbol of giving. Indeed, the earth teaches us that touching must take the place of taking, or the modern world will continue to destroy itself by devouring everything that is consumable.

EARTH RITUAL FOR HEALING ONE PERSON

The simplest earth rituals do not require great physical preparation. For example, imagine a person who is so caught up in an eating disorder that his inflated body makes him worry tremendously. Imagine also that this person is constantly trying to do things for others, to make them feel comfortable. An indigenous perception of this person is that he is using eating as a way to communicate his need for another type of nourishment—emotional nourishment. A group of people would gather around that person for an earth ritual. Each participant must know the person well. Together their knowledge of the person is complete.

At the start a prayer is made to the Great Mother to be present at the ritual. Each person is allowed to call on the Great Mother to help them summon the nurturer in themselves and to show them the way to give as much as they have to a person they care for very much. Then the person in need speaks about himself in prayerful terms, stressing that which constitutes the challenges in his life. It could sound something like this: "Oh, Great Mother, I come to you as a child very empty inside. I grew up in a family where I became the caretaker at very young age. I found myself trying to make things right for others. Never have I felt connected in ways that recognize my efforts. I feel as if I have never belonged to anything, and no matter how hard I work to correct this, my psyche suffers greatly from a silent ostracism. I'm tired of being a wanderer. I'm tired of giving that which I do not have. I'm tired of being told silently that this is all I can do. I want my real self to come out and to be seen. I want to go home, I want to be home. I want to be among people who see me for who I am, who make me feel as if I matter."

Such a prayer is somewhat general, but it contains enough emotional energy for the rest of the group to work with. The role of the group is now to address the person, one speaker at a time, praising everything that is good about him. This can be done in the form of a song, in plain words, or both. The goal is to make the person feel recognized, acknowledged, and alive. In order to do that, the group must demonstrate sincerity and great depth in their interaction with the person. Since a huge portion of human illness comes from not being seen, from the weight of anonymity upon the self, the purpose here is to remove the cloak of hiddenness from the person and to restore light to their psyche.

The amount of emotion released in this process can be enormous. One of the ways in which emotion is released is through touch. The way a person is held determines the amount of emotion released, and if words and hymns can be punctuated with sincere gestures of love, such as touch, the healing of the person can be very profound. Notice that this kind of ritual is supposed to focus entirely on one individual. Depending on how many people are present, the ritual can last from one to three hours.

This ritual can take place anywhere—in the living room of a house, in someone's backyard, or in an empty lecture room. Privacy in the open air would be best, but if that is not available in the modern world, a private, enclosed space will do. The earth part of the ritual is not the dirt or the sitting on the ground, but the words of acknowledgment and support, the collective attention to one person, and whenever possible the human touch. Because earth is support and attention, anytime we are positively spotlighted and feel great about it, we are receiving something earthy.

LYING ON THE EARTH'S LAP

The ritual called Lying on the Earth's Lap is one in which each individual rekindles her relationship with the earth. It allows the earth to absorb negative energy from our bodies. Therefore, a person who is ill, who has been the victim of abuse, who feels burned out, who is lonely, and who cannot connect should consider this type of ritual. Similarly, a person who is constantly surrounded by scarcity, who feels that nothing exciting is happening in her life, whose relationship is falling apart, or who has experienced a recent loss should also try this ritual.

Usually, the ritual takes place at a large shrine made of earth, either built as a platform or as a large mound, surrounded with a variety of foods. A well-defined gateway marks the entrance to the shrine. There is always another area, separate from the ritual space, well defined and distinguished by a fire at its center, which serves as the village. From there people go to the earth shrine and release their emotion to the Great Mother, then return to the village, where they are cheerfully welcomed. The container of the village is held together by the dynamics of rhythm and chant. (A container in ritual language is an activity that is meant to keep the energy focused. Chanting and drumming often keep people's attention affixed to what is going on.) In it people dance with one another and sing together, united by the persistent, regular drumbeat.

At the earth shrine, which is guarded at the gate by keepers and at the shrine itself by healers, the mood is a little bit different. As each person arrives at the gate, he or she is greeted by the gatekeepers who tell them what is about to happen. Each person is reminded that their purpose in going to the shrine is to vigorously communicate to the Earth Mother that which has been the source of trouble in their life. They are told to come into intimate contact with the earth by lying on her lap like a trusting and vulnerable baby in a loving mother's arms. Then the individual is escorted by the gatekeeper to the shrine, where he is passed to the healers. The healers reiterate what the gatekeepers have said, with encouragement not to hold back from the Earth Mother. The goal is to keep the individual constantly reminded of the depth of what he or she is about to do, and to be as specific as possible about the nature of the problems that they are bringing to offer to the Earth Mother.

As mediators, the healers must stand by discreetly to give any additional help the individual may need. More often than not, sacred contact with the earth results in a tremendous surge of emotion. The healers make sure they maintain some kind of physical contact with the person throughout the ritual so that there is a constant sense of reinforcement from the village through them.

The time required for the healing depends on individual needs. There is no way to regulate the amount of time a person stays with the earth, as it depends on how much emotional unloading is needed. When the person's healing is complete, the healers escort the individual to the gatekeepers, who take him back to the village. Now at the village are a few people on the lookout for the returning villager. When they see him coming, they scream the villager's name, attracting the attention of everyone. As the person enters the village he is received with hugs and cheers. In Dagara, people say that we must learn from dogs how to welcome one another, because our dogs are masters at making us feel wanted. It is not infrequent to hear people say, "Give him a dog's-style welcome." While the returning villager is being cared for by the village, another villager leaves for the shrine. This ritual lasts as long as there are people to be healed.

A RITUAL OF SYMBOLIC BURIAL

The above two rituals, however emotionally radical they are, do not match in intensity one that consists of a literal confinement of the self in the earth. Sometimes referred to as taking cover under the earth, or as a burial ritual, this is one of the earth rituals in which people return symbolically into the earth's womb and, inside the earth, experience being reshaped for a possible rebirth. Two postures are available in this case, either horizontal confinement or vertical confinement. In horizontal confinement, people are buried while lying flat. In vertical confinement, they are buried in an upright position.

Standard initiation practices involve vertical burial. The initiate is buried from the neck down overnight. The feeling is hard to describe, but similar to a paralysis; you feel yourself connected to a body that you can't move. The other strong perception is that you are very close to the earth, as if you are a quite small being. Your whole height above ground is the height of your head. The insight you get after the first hour is extremely fascinating. It feels like everything is very close by, and that you are a remarkably small entity in the universe. But as you stay in this posture long enough, there is a feeling of being held together by someone. If you go into dream time or a trance state, you might see light everywhere and loud noises that are not, however, frightening. If you are a claustrophobic, you might experience the opposite. A six-hour confinement will make you feel like you are being dismantled, cut into pieces. But then you move into a deeply peaceful state.

People should be allowed to choose which kind of confinement suits them. Vertical confinement requires digging deep into the earth, as opposed to horizontal confinement, which works with shallow trenches. Usually the people expected to participate in the ritual must prepare the ritual space themselves. Their job is to create a cemetery in a few hours, which they decorate and make beautiful. For this they can use flowers, ferns, branches, anything that suits their imagination. Next to the cemetery is the village area, where people will drum, sing, and dance.

The actual burials of people take place simultaneously when there are enough holes for half of the village involved in the ritual. One person buries another person, then returns to the village space to sing, drum, and dance. The buried ones are cared for by a small team of keepers for the duration of time they stay confined in the earth. When they are uncovered, the other group will take their places. A six-hour ritual, with a three-hour burial for each individual, is typical. The choreographic design of the ritual depends on the people doing the ritual. However it must include an invocation with some prayers to the great spirit of the earth and to the ancestors whose bodies remain indefinitely in earth confinement, a prayer intended to help make the ritual a true rebirth for everyone. At the end of the ritual, there must be an opportunity for the village to send praises to the Earth Mother for the wonderful feeling of being reborn.

People usually experience this ritual as a combination of pain and tremendous vision. As the body remains trapped in the earth, the person's spirit is freed after a painful struggle through an imaginary birth canal. Some people describe it as a long and suffocating tunnel that ends in light and great vision. At the end of the tunnel is great relief and a feeling of freedom. But people must stay inside the earth long enough, and endure the pain of confinement sufficiently, to break into this state. This is why this kind of experience is not for everybody and should not be tried just for curiosity's sake.

There is a ritual similar to the burial ritual described above involving burial in liquid earth. This ritual is different from merely being bathed in mud. Though they share the same purpose, which is to allow the earth to absorb any poison that the body holds, the mud-bath ritual has the softness and the gentleness of the touch of a human hand and is quite nurturing. The intention of the liquid earth burial ritual is pointed toward release, not nourishment. The purpose is to get rid of the toxins that accumulate as a result of the multitude of human addictions and to free the body from them. The mixture of water and earth, the two principal elements in the wheel, provides a means of flooding the negative energies in the body and flushing them out into the earth.

The most effective way to understand the mud-burial ritual is to look at the process symbolically. It is a way to return to a state where one becomes more receptive to positive nourishment. This presupposes that good nourishment cannot be received by people full of the toxins of negativity. Most of the time people do not even recognize the presence of such poison. The release of bad things, known or unknown, allows the freed self to receive good things.

To do this, it is best to establish an arrangement much like those I have already described, including a village place and a healing place. We have described the village as a place held together by chant, fire, and rhythm. People will exit or enter it through a gateway. The healing place in this case will be an area where people's bodies are covered with wet earth. It must be carefully prepared to have the look of a healing place, and attractive enough to motivate people to go there. It must be staffed by at least two healers, people with knowledge of how to help a person's psyche by means of words and touch. These people are key to the success of this ritual. They must communicate to each villager a deep understanding of the seriousness of what they are doing. The whole experience must not feel as if one were getting dirty.

The healers are helped by two gatekeepers who, as each villager exits the village place for the journey to healing, prepare him through careful words of explanation and encouragement. By the time the villager has been escorted to the healing place, the villager is well prepared to surrender to the process and to release whatever emotion is held inside. When the healing is completed, the villager must be handed over to an escort, who will then accompany him back to the village area. It is, as always, important to give a person a warm welcome home upon their return from a healing session.

At this juncture, it feels to me that earth rituals are those that Westerners need most to reduce the sense of isolation and increase their sense of belonging. The rituals described above can be adapted to fit the needs of any group. They can be done as regularly as needed until there is a sense of unity within the group. There is so much in human beings that needs rejuvenating that these kinds of ritual cannot be abused. If these rituals are done properly with co-workers, for instance, they could increase people's productivity, reduce the number of crises, and allow people truly to make their home in their workplaces.

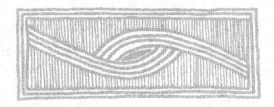

13.

Mineral Rituals

The stones have given me music
that figures for me their holes in the earth
and their long lying in the dark.
—WENDELL BERRY, from "The Stones"

Mineral rituals aim at restoring lost memories. We have described the element mineral as the storage place of information and have explained that when there is a break in continuity of information and history, society experiences turbulence. One of the key memories that mineral rituals evoke is the life purpose linked to each human being. As I have said, in many indigenous cultures, it is understood that everyone comes into this world for a reason. In order to enter into this world, one must have an approved project to carry out. The problem is that the clarity with which we embark on our journey to earth begins to fade upon arrival. Our ability to accomplish our purpose requires a village in which there are other people who know what our purpose is and are able to design a system that presents us with continual reminders of it throughout our lives.

Everyone is gifted. This means that everyone has something to give. A person who does not feel gifted is lost in a pit of oblivion and confusion. Sometimes we are the last people to recognize our own gifts. When they are shown to us by a group of people, they carry a different and larger meaning, and we feel acknowledged and recognized, which increases our sense of belonging. The task of a community is to use its knowledge of each person's gifts to help the person make a connection between his or her gifts and the images of strength that regularly occur in that person's psyche. In this way each person can then act from the knowledge of her or his unique purpose. In other words, we are born with a profession, and to be most proficient as we go through life, all we need to do is remember our profession.

MINERAL RITUALS AND IDENTITY CRISES

A person's purpose is energetically inscribed in their bones and its actual translation into work should agree with the message engraved in these bones. The question is, what happens when what you do does not align with who you are? It means that you are betraying the very vitality that defines you and are thus inviting great pain into your life. You are likely to experience low self-worth, a lack of enthusiasm about what you are doing, and, above all, of a nagging sense of inner emptiness. In short, you will experience an identity crisis.

So many people in the modern world, caught between their commitment to survival and their intuitive allegiance to a genuine life purpose, find themselves forced to sacrifice their purpose to make a living. It is for these people that mineral rituals must be done. Their very livelihood undermines their reason for being. There is no greater harm done to a person than the harm of a life activity that competes against, or contradicts, their purpose. The modern world does not seem to provide an ideal place for people to pursue their life project, for the very survival of the Western economic system demands a state of constant striving and sacrifice from the people who work within it. It may seem that you are threatening your economic survival if you abandon the prevailing economic system to pursue something as seemingly intangible as a personal life purpose. Yet pursuing one's life purpose is the foundation on which the health of both the individual and the community rests.

Indigenous people know that there is collective memory and there is individual memory. Collective memory is not a vast well that exists separate from individual people. It is the sum total of the personal memories of each person. In other words, for a village, a tribe, and a culture to remember, each individual must master the ability to remember the knowledge that lives in his or her bones.

Indigenous people recognize that when the individual does not remember, gradually it is the culture, the society, that forgets. Individuals who forget their life purpose put the whole community at risk. They begin to look outside themselves for their purpose, and society often responds to their demand by creating artificial goals. But society loses in this process, because it is not receiving what is the individual's to give. Not to know what gift you're bringing to your people implies that you cannot deliver. If you cannot give, it means that the community cannot receive from you.

STONE AND MINERAL RITUALS AMONG THE DAGARA

The first time I encountered a stone in a ritual sense was in the course of my initiation. We were on the last few days of a six-week-long series of journeys. This last journey was to the Other World. I had reached that place after crawling inside a cave. I was supposed to bring something back from the Other World, but I had not been told specifically what that thing was supposed to be. Looking down, I glimpsed a stone. The stone attracted me because it was unusually shiny. It was like a breathing star that opened and closed. When I picked it up, I was thrown into a strange dream world, an experience that culminated with my feeling that I was inside the very stone I was holding. The stone had grown bigger and bigger right in front of me. Once inside, I had a series of epiphanies that took me back several lifetimes. My memory was working with graphic accuracy. When I was released by the stone, it stopped shining. I brought the stone back with me to the everyday world. It has never left me since.

My experience with the stone in initiation shows the property of stones and minerals to stimulate memory. Since then I have needed to be reminded of their power. Even with a special stone, it is possible to forget! The following story shows how a member of my village community helped me remember a part of my purpose through a stone ritual.

A few years ago a diviner in my village told me that a spirit from the past had grafted itself onto me and had to be acknowledged and integrated for my own good. The diviner pointed at me, saying, "This spirit will help your memory, and you will find words in your work to communicate what needs to be said."

I did not take his words seriously. After all, diviners, who can see things ordinary people can't, might just possibly be seeing something that isn't really there! So I dismissed his statement on this ground.

The diviner pointed to a stone and began explaining that I needed to do a ritual acknowledging whatever it was that had grafted itself onto me. He said, "You will find a stone. When you do, bring it to the family shrine and leave it there after making a prayer in which you state why you are bringing this stone to this sacred place. After three days, you will bring food, water, and a bottle of liquor. Make the same prayer again, but add a request for nourishment, both for this spirit and for you. Then wait and see what happens to you."

Still feeling skeptical, I asked how I was supposed to find the stone. He reproached me for not believing in him and said I would in a few days if I did what he asked. He then added, "In the course of one of the next three nights, you will step on the stone that you are supposed to find. You will know it because the experience will be quite memorable. If stepping on it still does not make you believe in it, don't do the ritual, throw that stone away, and come back, and I will tell you what else will happen."

The image of stepping on a stone stuck with me, and I decided that I would be careful for the next three days. I paid great attention to every step I was taking, making sure I knew where I was putting my feet. It was nerve-racking. I felt paranoid. How could stepping on a stone be memorable enough to convince me that the stone came from Spirit? After the first twenty-four hours, my nerves were shot. I decided I should try to relax, for if this was supposed to happen, it would, no matter how much or how little attention I gave to it. I then felt a little better. Nothing happened the next day or the next night. I became more confident that the diviner was just trying to upset my self-assuredness. Still I had one more day and night to go, so I remained somewhat vigilant.

The last night, I decided to stay indoors all the time rather than risk tripping over a rock. If I had to go out to use the bathroom, I would take two flashlights with me. Then I went to sleep and had bad dreams that I could not recall. I woke up before dawn feeling very strange. It was then that I decided that this diviner had indeed lied to me and had put me through three days and nights of discomfort for nothing. They were over, and now I had to go tell him how I felt.

The rays from the still-unrisen sun made it quite easy to move around without flashlight. I decided to go out and greet the sunrise. No sooner had I taken my second step toward the doorway than I bumped my toes against something hard. The shock of the impact was so unexpected that I lost my balance and would have crashed on the floor if I hadn't been close enough to the door to hang on to it. Two of my toenails were shattered, and blood was streaming out. When I had recovered slightly from the pain, I looked on the ground, and there was a red rock the size of two fists put together. The impact with my foot had rolled it about two feet closer to the door. My first thought was that someone had placed it here while I was asleep. Cursing, I took the rock outside. The sun had already risen, but no one was out yet. I dropped the rock in a secure place and took care of my wound, then carried the rock to the "infamous" diviner. My mood was not good.

He smiled when he saw me come. I told him I wanted some explanation. He asked if I had done what I was supposed to do upon tripping over the stone. I could tell he knew I had not done it. He refused to give me another consultation, and I left in a state of confusion.

Back home, I brought the stone to the family shrine and made my prayers. The next three days were quiet and peaceful in comparison to the previous paranoid days. I felt like a different person. Some energy was in me that hadn't been there before. I could feel it. On the third day I brought offerings of food and water and a bottle of liquor produced locally. I told the story of my encounter with the rock in a long, detailed prayer, including everything the diviner had advised me to say. Then I added that I just wanted to stay out of trouble and if doing this would help, so be it. That day, my belief in stones deepened. I continued to feel as if some new ability to communicate had taken root in me, and this increased ability has helped me in living out my purpose of communicating from the deep memories of my people. For reasons such as these, rituals of mineral and stone will be helpful also to Western people.

A MINERAL RITUAL FOR REMEMBERING

A basic ritual for remembering begins with the premise that we are alienated from our purpose and that society, in turn, is alienated from its purpose. First a shrine for the ritual must be made of stones and bones. These stones and bones should come from many sources and be as diverse as possible. This diversity is representative of the diversity of purposes. Just as modern cemeteries are crowded with stones, each one representing the memory of a dead person, the gathered stones of the mineral ritual represent the memory lying within the individuals gathered at the shrine. The bones represent the stones of the body. The arrangement of the stones and bones depends on the ingenuity of the people in charge of the shrine. As we have mentioned for other shrines, there should be an easily identified point of entrance, representing a gateway into the sacred space of the shrine. Overall the ritual space will look as though it has a nucleus that contains all these objects and a plasma, which is the space around the objects where people are going to assemble. This center place is the place of memory. In contrast, the outer space is the place where supportive forces are built and forwarded to the center. The building of this energy happens in rhythm and chant.

The ritual itself must focus on individuals, whose task is to remember moments in their lives when they felt strong, connected, powerful, and useful, moments when the world around them seemed like a true home, familiar and welcoming. Everyone has moments like this; even if they are faint or short-lived, they constitute a window through which we briefly see the possibility of our realignment with our purpose. With the group gathered together, each person holds a stone in his or her hand and listens for images, thoughts, and impressions to surface. The energy of stone is allowed to awaken memories within. After a period of time, which is determined by how fluent people are in listening to the messages of mineral, a sharing will follow. The listening process involves the locking of one's mind and spirit onto the stone and a letting go of any control or distraction. If this step can be achieved, graphic images will stream in. This indicates that an interaction is in progress. Each person describes to the group the images that most frequently came to consciousness during the listening period. The images are symbolic of the purpose to which each person is linked. This presentation of images allows the rest of the group to reflect upon these images and to understand the person's unique qualities and gifts.

At the end of the ritual, the group will pray for the discovered memories to be kept alive, illuminating our path in the dark routes of our journey. People are urged to retain in their awareness what they have remembered. This sharing ritual is usually lengthy, but it provides the initial material to allow people to begin thinking about their areas, places and times of strength.

STORYTELLING AS A MINERAL RITUAL

In the village stories are clearly seen as in the domain of the element mineral, holding the key to memory and purpose. Everyone must participate and bathe in mythologies. Stories are not just for children; they are for the child in everyone, who remembers and understands. Stories open a world wherein relating to others and the world is automatic, and they boost imagination toward a place of better self-knowledge. Without stories, a society will find it difficult to hold itself together. It is as if stories bond people together and allow each individual to better comprehend what their place is in the world, and how their place holds everything else together. Indigenous teachings are derived from stories that they see as eternal blueprints for human wisdom. Like a forest in which countless beings find their home, stories are places where each one of us can find a home. The home in the story is the image we hang on to and identify with. It represents our address in the city of the story. This home can change from story to story and from one day to the next. This is because as the circumstances of our lives change, so too does the place we inhabit in stories.

In ritual storytelling, the narrative must guide and inspire people. First the story must be chosen to reflect current matters. Then someone must tell it in a way that involves every listener, so that everyone finds something to identify with in the story, and the teller and audience become one. The teller borrows his story from the pool of ancestral lore. As they listen, people must find a place for themselves inside the story. This place will be each person's area of focus as they work to recall their deep identity. Who we are appears spontaneously within myth if we allow ourselves to be open to it. Each place in the story is a milestone representing someone, and everyone's position in the story will be more or less different.

At the end of the story, each person should have received some further insight into his or her own purpose or position. Such clarity indicates an ability to locate oneself even in the middle of chaos and confusion. It is as if confusion and dissatisfaction are the psyche's way of telling us that we're not where we're supposed to be. Clarity about one's position is essential to our sense of identity and important for healing because ritual storytelling can be of great value in helping people locate themselves in society and in the world.

A STORY

My mother loved music and would always sing a story to me when we had to walk any great distance. She would make up the song in the process of telling me the story. The story was usually about some unfortunate girl or woman, usually an orphan. One I remember in particular, related previously in *Of Water and the Spirit*, was about a girl named Kula, whose mother died and left her with a little sister, Naab, to take to their aunt. Kula loved to dress well. So while Woor, her slave, packed, she dressed herself as the queen she was. When they were ready to go, the slave girl had packed a lot of water, while Kula only carried her little sister, Naab. After walking for some time, Kula felt thirsty and asked for water. Woor traded a little water for one of Kula's gold rings. The heat of the day encouraged thirst, and Woor was the only supplier of water to Naab and Kula. So the exchange went on and on, until the slave girl was dressed up like a queen, and Kula, stripped of her finery, looked like a slave. As they neared their destination, Kula was tired of carrying her little sister, and so Woor, who looked now like a queen, offered to carry Naab.

When the trio arrived at the aunt's house, the aunt couldn't tell who was who. She thought that Woor was the queen since she had all the gold on her, and Kula looked very much like the slave. And so it was that Woor and Naab were welcomed into the royal family, while Kula, with nothing to prove that she was a princess, was treated as a slave and sent out to guard the crops against wild animals.

People who guard crops must sing to keep animals away. Kula sang, but it was more like a sad cry for her mistaken identity and a prayer for help to the beings of the wild. One day the *kontombli*, the spirits who live in the underworld, were passing by. Her mournful voice fell gently into the listening ears of these beings as they held their breaths to take in the whole story. Because she was telling the truth, and the *kontombli* knew it because they are superior, they said to her, "Go home, little lady. Your troubles are over. Your aunt's eyes will be opened, and she will know who you are."

When Kula arrived home, her aunt recognized her at once as her true niece. Her identity was restored, and her aunt felt remorse that she had not recognized her. The slave girl was sent out immediately to guard the crops. She could not sing because she had a bad voice that sent out horrible sounds when she tried to sing. Along came a different group of *kontombli*. They had come to listen to the farm girl's enchanting voice. They asked, "We heard that your voice brings tears to the heart. Please let us hear that song you sing every day."

Woor did not have manners and knew nothing about what Kula had experienced, so she replied rudely, "What are you talking about? I ain't got no song to sing to nobody." Then she emitted some raucous sounds, which, to the sensitive ears of *kontombli*, sounded like the smell of vomit.

Disgusted and puzzled, they asked Woor once more for a real song. Answering their courtesy with rudeness, the girl rebuked them in the same way. Believing they had been deceived by the girl, the *kontombli* grew so angry that they turned her to stone.

As the narrative ends, people have either seen themselves as the slave girl, the queen, or the little sister. Some people may even have identified with the *kontombli*. If someone identifies with the slave girl, the indigenous would say that such a person was in his past life a slave, and has returned to heal the wounds of slavery. If someone feels attracted to the queen image, this is because that person's gifts are about to blossom, and it is time to give them greater attention. Identifying with the beings from the other side is interpreted similarly to identification with the queen. However, there is a touch of spiritual genius in such a person. Therefore, the way to tell who could be open to a spiritual path is informed partly by this attraction. It is almost impossible for a story to leave some people out. As we enter a story, we are invited to join that which in the story is the closest extension of who we are and the process we are involved with.

The healing dimension of this story is the revelation of where one is in the story. To the indigenous, healing has a lot to do with knowing where you are in your life journey. What the story heals is precisely the dark spots in people's lives that are pointed out to them by the story. Thus, for someone who relates to the queen, the knowing that this means to await consciously the blossoming of one's gift will help one move in the right direction.

To begin to appreciate stories as healing tools and not merely as entertainment or information, a simple first step is to begin asking of a story, "Where am I in it? What or whom do I identify with?" A little imagination will help discern the cosmological meaning of it.

The reason fiction dealing with the supernatural is so attractive in the West is that it echoes in the bones the need to become more acquainted with the world of the spirit. The Other World is precisely the world that in the West has been forgotten. This attraction is memory itself arising, pulled out of its dormant state by imaginary forms. The attraction that Halloween has for Americans, the popularity of horror films and stories, all point to a place within that is resisting total obliteration. Behind these tales, wrestling for a place to live, are countless memories that have been frozen in the cells of people's bones. These memories can be fully awakened only in the context of ritual. As a result, every ritual performed in the West is a wake-up call to memories hidden in people. Some of these memories deeply disturb their recipients, who know no way to manage them. Other images add a powerful new dimension to their recipients' lives. This is why every mineral ritual must include a period of listening, for listening is the complement of storytelling.

MINERAL, MEMORY, AND COLLECTIONS

Westerners often respond to what they hear their bones telling them by collecting and storing various objects. To the indigenous, watching the objects a person collects provides a clue to what spiritual source a person is drawn toward. For example, there is a young man in my maternal family who, after his father died, began acting quite unusually. Not only was he speaking out loud by himself most of the time, refusing human companionship, but he was also quite inexplicably collecting scraps of metal. The little room he occupied in the compound was crowded with random metal objects, from bicycle parts to old tin cans, radio antennae, and dead lightbulbs taken from flashlights. From these pieces of scrap he made things that appeared to be almost functional.

He would sit alone quietly as if listening to an inner voice, then make a sound of agreement before picking up an item from his junk pile, then listen some more while looking around. It was obvious that he was being instructed by Spirit about what to collect and what to do with the things he collected. The results were sometimes amazing. He was the first in the village to build a shortwave radio—instructed only by Spirit—and he designed a system of electronic circuitry to make his room into a symphony of flashing lights. He would spend his day mostly listening to the Other World, reporting on what he heard on any subject.

Healers gathered around him and performed a ritual reconciliation, which allowed him not only to continue making his strange machines, but also, and more important, to use his gift to help other people in need. He has perfected an ability to listen to what the Spirit says about someone and then to translate the message verbatim to that person. He has become, in a sense, a radio transmitter for the world of Spirit.

This boy's instinct to collect was prompted by the Other World in such a way that it became an almost priestly gesture. To respond sincerely to the urging of a voice within, and in such a way that it serves the greatest good, is to become a priest of some sort. Even in the modern world, where collecting is understood as appropriation and consumption, it is nevertheless prompted by a message from the deep. The urge to collect is the natural response of the human psyche to an aesthetic object that speaks directly to it, stirring memories that lie deeply within. Collecting confirms the indigenous belief that the human psyche reads and understands symbols and that the attraction to beauty is a function of psychic awareness.

I think museums are born out of the West's confused response to things that speak directly to the psyche. How else can one explain the widespread presence of sacred indigenous art, particularly African art, in the West? African artistic productions are more accessible outside of Africa than inside it. In some stores and museums, it is often frightening to view live ancestral masks displayed as if their purpose and function were to be looked at. These objects emit powerful energies because they are alive. Westerners do not realize that they are being affected by the energy put out by these live sacred objects. In Africa, a person who knows and understands the dynamic between art and culture will run away when he confronts living but displaced masks. For the person who remembers, a statue representing the ancestors or the Spirit World invokes energies that only a dedicated priest can handle.

The West's attraction to collecting icons from the rest of the world seems, to indigenous people, not only a symptom of its disconnection from the past but also an instinctive yet unfocused response to a confused memory that is speaking too loudly for the psyche to ignore. The good part in this is that Western memory is being jogged by contact with the powerful objects from other parts of the world. The bad part is that people who flirt with powerful objects from the past are playing with energies they don't know how to interact with. They should first understand their attraction in terms of a deeply hidden ancestral pull that finds its reflection in the object. This attraction is the beginning of their awakening to their deep spiritual self, perhaps even their real self. It is also a response to the call of the Other World.

To further the awakening begun by attraction to a symbolic object, frame your attraction in a series of ritual dialogues in which you speak to the things you are attracted to. In this dialogue, it is important to speak to the object as though it is animated by a spirit and is alive, not as though it is simply a symbolic representation of something in the distance. In the indigenous view, a mask of an ancestor is not a symbol of the ancestor, it *is* the ancestor. An indigenous person, upon hearing that the mask is only a carving, not the spirit itself, may well respond coldly that this means the speaker can't see. The eye of the indigenous sees a lot more than appearance.

Then, as you engage in dialogue with the object, describe to it as clearly as possible the feelings and images that arise in you as you associate with the object. Such an exercise means recognizing that to be attracted to ancestral objects is to be called by another world. The attraction is an invitation to respond, whether or not one knows exactly how to proceed. The simple acknowledgment of having heard the call is enough.

Mineral tells us that we know what we need to know, if we would but remember. In our bones is the knowledge that tells us how to connect to the ancestral energies through the fire, how to decipher the hieroglyphics of nature, how to nourish ourselves from the abundance of the earth without destroying it, and how to find reconciliation to a myriad of troubles and woes in the water. Mineral is also metal, the wire of communication that connects all of the individuals in a community through stories and collective memories. The elders say that the rocks can speak, but their voice is so tiny that it can barely be heard. The rocks remind us to be still and to listen carefully, to stop searching outside of ourselves for that which we already hold within.

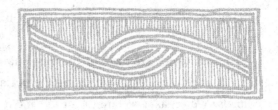

14.

Nature Rituals

. . . each pond with its blazing lilies
is a prayer heard and answered
—MARY OLIVER, "Morning Poem"

Healer and medicine man Eliot Cowan, in his book *Plant Spirit Medicine*, remarks that the most striking thing about our relationship with plants is that we need them but they don't need us. We humans are utterly dependent on plants to cover all our needs: fuel, shelter, clothing, medicine, the petrochemical cornucopia, and, of course, food. In contrast, plant communities do just fine without people. We seem to offer nothing but suffering, destruction, and the threat of extinction.

Human beings are most of the time unaware of the extent and intimacy of their connection with nature, especially the world of plants and animals. We act as if we are the proud and dominant other and thus can and should manifest our superiority in ways that are rather careless and devastating to nature. Indeed, trees live in harmony, and we create dissonance. Yet we want to live in a world where everyone and everything is harmoniously linked to everyone and to everything. It is the project of nature rituals and the nature people among us to reaffirm continuously this interdependence.

It is hard to separate nature rituals from water, fire, earth, and mineral rituals. Since every ritual is an attempt to change our relationship with the Other World, and since nature is all about change and transformation, there is some sense in which every ritual pertains to nature and aims to reveal, heal, and reinstate our own innermost nature.

NATURE RITUALS AND PURPOSE

Nature rituals, like mineral rituals, help people remain focused on their true purpose. To be human is to be engaged in a challenging task of continual readjustment and fine-tuning, especially in a world that struggles to distance itself from nature. The repeated distractions that plague life in the modern world separate us not only from the natural world but from our own essential nature.

The modern world is a denaturalized world that regards nature as something standing in the way of progress. Consequently, people need nature rituals in order to get closer to their inner selves and to nature. Any one of the rituals described thus far can combine nature with its principal element. Doing so is as simple as making sure that the place you choose for the ritual is as close to nature as possible. Indeed, while it is possible to do a ritual in an amphitheater or in a hotel ballroom, this same ritual will generate greater energy if done in the woods. In the modern world, as in the indigenous world, ritual is best done out-of-doors, surrounded by the elements of the natural world.

A NATURE RITUAL WITH TREES

My first nature ritual, as I related in chapter 2, consisted of looking at a tree. The exercise led me to change my attitude toward trees. It made me realize how much patient love and caring a tree can have. It allowed me to grasp more fully the concept of trees as our guardians, commissioned by our Mother the earth to provide safety and comfort as we travel through life.

Let us take a group of people willing to explore nature and the trees ritualistically, and let us guide them through the process. We cannot assume that these people live in nature. Therefore, in the morning of the ritual, they should gather for an invocation in which they brief the spirit of nature on what is about to happen. In their prayer an emphasis should be placed on homecoming, recognizing in words the long separation, which has caused so much loss. A humble request should be made for guidance as to how to look, how to notice, how to acknowledge what is noticed. The prayer should explain to Spirit and to the ritual participants that we are going to walk inside the bosom of nature. While we wander silently, we will listen for a calling from a tree. If and when we do feel called, we will go sit and be with the tree that called us long enough to experience communion with it.

After the prayer people can silently walk into the woods and wander separately until each one of them finds a tree that calls. The idea is to sit on the earth facing the tree that called to you, and meditate with it. This means deleting any mental activity that distracts from being present to the tree. Meanwhile, somewhere in the woods an elder or a ritual leader will play a drum, slowly and gently sending sound waves to every station where a person is interacting with a tree. After several hours have passed, the ritual leader begins chanting, and everyone will know that it is time to go where the voice comes from. It may take another hour or two for everyone to return. A closing prayer of acknowledgment and gratitude for what has happened is in order. Then people can gather back at a designated place where they can spend some time sharing what they experienced in the woods.

NATURE AND FIRE

In every village and tribal community, the nights are challenged for a little while by bonfires, around which stories are told and retold. People go to sleep wrapped in the blanket of long and endless, warm stories. The dream world and images that these stories take us into are quite unique. Because these stories often involve beings from the Other World intermingling with people in the village among the trees and plants of nature, there is a continued sense of warm and purposeful intimacy in them. The wood that burns is nature releasing its fire so that people can continue to shine even in their sleep.

When the sun goes to sleep, nature awakens with magic and mystery that puts the psyche on its toes. More than anything else, the fire that is released by nature for our good is the fire that bonds people together. It is the community heartbeat reaffirming harmony. It is why they say that love and respect cannot live long without periodic reheating at the fireplace of nature. When we are intimately connected with the natural world, the heart that beats inside of us echoes the vibration out there and warms us up with vitality. Otherwise when there is no fire to keep the psyche fed with symbolism, people will turn cold even before they go to sleep. A cold heart fosters stale dreams and steals excitement from life. Thus the burning fire at night is symbolic of the awakening of nature and our nature, joining hands to provide greater richness to our lives.

Here is a short but lively nature ritual with fire: It requires a blazing bonfire, people, some animal costumes and body paint, and some rhythm. In this ritual participants will pick an animal, or a being from the wild, whose dance they will mimic. The ritual is similar to carnivals, which, when done properly, are nature rituals where animals often play a large role. In a carnival setting, such as Mardi Gras and many other celebrations practiced throughout the West, people may get the chance to do the dance of a particular animal. In this mimetic behavior, the inner child is awakened. Like a child who hasn't yet learned to wear a mask, one gets in touch with the natural magic that one carries.

When this ritual is done in Africa, a totem animal is usually the animal picked. Among countless tribal communities in Africa, every person has an animal correspondence, called a totem animal. This is an animal with whom the person has a special kinship, and therefore the animal provides a frame of reference in the quest for change. In other words, your identity is the same as the identity of your totem animal. If you lose track of your identity, you have the totem animal to remind you of it.

You do not need to live in an indigenous village to claim a totem animal. To find your totem animal, observe your dreams for the type of animal that appears in them. Also keep an eye on what creatures you encounter when you are in nature. It is not difficult for an attentive person to learn these things.

To prepare for the ritual, each participant picks an animal with whom she or he has a special kinship and then dresses accordingly. If you pick a lion, you must find a way to become a lion, either by painting yourself or by wearing a lion's hide. The less recognizable you are as a human and the closer you are to your animal, the better. Once dressed as animals, participants are stationed all around the bonfire, looking otherworldly and very colorful.

A ritual leader opens the ritual by leading everyone in an invocation, inviting nature and its inhabitants to partake in this moment of communication with our true nature. The invocation may sound like this: "Beings from the wilds, ancestors, spirits of nature, we invoke your leadership among us, that each one of us may see himself or herself using the eyes with which you see the world. Take over our bodies that we may move as you do in the elegance and beauty of healing."

Then rhythm and chant take over, and the dance begins. At first it appears to be a free-for-all, with everyone parading around the fire. But this warm-up period soon turns into a display, in which every represented nature dweller shows everyone else what he or she's got. The ritual leader calls the name of an animal, usually preceding the animal's name with the attribute "brother" or "sister." Hence you can hear something like, "Brother lion, king of the realm, speak." Or "Sister turtle, who's smart enough to carry your home around, give us a treat." Every time someone is called, the person is supposed to dance his or her way into the circle and to formally parade in rhythm for a few minutes while absorbing the attention of the group.

The healing in this ritual comes from becoming the other, the totem animal. Doing so will send away the spirits of illness, for in becoming the animal, each dancer changes himself or herself, and the resulting unfamiliar energy structure drives out the spirit of illness. That is, in the mind of the indigenous, illness is like an unwelcome guest that wants the place it has taken over to remain the same so that it can be comfortable. Certain healing practices, such as this one, involve altering the energy structure of the person. By doing this, the illness, if there is any, becomes "irritated" at the rude hospitality and moves away in search of another place. The animal one chooses to become represents the powers that one wishes to bring out into the world. In the village this ritual is done yearly at the end of the farming season and at the start of the hunting season.

At the end of the ritual, the ritual leader thanks each being from the wild who participated in this moment of intensity and brings the ritual to a close. Usually after the formal closure people return to free-for-all dancing until dawn.

NATURE AND WATER

For the Dagara people, the rain goddess, Sapla, is a tree. She is soaked with water, and should she dry up, there will be no rain for seven years. The roots of the tree and the plant are veins and arteries needing clean and nourishing water, which is sent upward to the rest of the body. This water must be pure, it must be real water, or it will not work. Our constitution functions just the same way. The heart needs to pump clean water out and across to the rest of the body. We can't pollute that water with chemicals, or we will suffer a long nightmare of turmoil and illness.

The rainmaker in traditional Africa is the intermediary between the people and the rain goddess, who is the life giver of the community. Pollution of the waterways, or even of the ground, dries up the rain tree, puts the rainmaker out of work, and sends the land and the tribe into years and years of drought. Pollution of ourselves sends a confusing image to the rain goddess, and the transformation of our contaminated veins and arteries becomes reflected in the gradual depletion of nature. We pollute ourselves when we act in ways that are not healing to us. Thus the blood and the water of human arteries must maintain a strict purity to give us the natural vitality we deserve.

Here is an example of a ritual self-decontamination. It is a ritual in which people shouldn't mind getting wet. It can happen almost anywhere, but the ideal place should be at a stream. The participants each get a branch of a tree, a plant, or a piece of stone. Plants and stones do not pollute the waterways. In fact, they purify water by filtering and retaining certain impurities. Participants stand together and face the stream, which has been carefully decorated with all sorts of plants and flowers. The ritual leader prays to the nature spirit to come running into our veins and arteries with the intention of cleaning up impurities that have entered us. The spirit of nature is asked to join hands with the spirit of water in the great cleansing job that we owe to ourselves. The leader stresses that the group cannot do this on its own and insists that every clumsy gesture be turned into a sacred purifying act that brings everyone closer to the beauty and bounty of Mother Nature.

After the invocation, people begin chanting. Meanwhile the leader, assisted by a few other people, goes to the stream. One after the other, people walk to the stream, and the facilitators rain water on them with the branches that the participants have brought. They return soaked but reverent about the manner in which water was brought to them by nature. After the last person goes through, the facilitators do the same thing to each other, then join the rest of the group for a closing prayer. As usual, this prayer acknowledges and thanks the spirits for what they have made possible. It will stress that this cleansing will show up in the days to come in the way each person lives his or her daily life.

The problem here in the West is that a great number of streams are polluted and need cleansing before they can actually participate in cleansing us. In this case a ritual must be done to heal pollution and waterways. It will take the form of a give-away of something nourishing to us. Because it does not have to be put into the water, and in any case is not a significant amount, the give-away can be any natural item, from food and fruit to tobacco and incense. Participants will gather at the appointed place at the waterfront, each one holding their give-away. The ritual leader will attract everyone's attention to the invocation, by speaking about what our own ignorance, greed, and carelessness have done to our nature. He or she will stress that we are here first to confess and then to try to repair what we've done wrong. In order for this to work out well, we need to call on every power from the Other World we know to help us find a proper way to atone. The leader will give room to every participant to invite a spirit ally who might help him or her be honest and open at this time in order for this healing to happen.

After the opening prayer, people will begin singing a lament song. Meanwhile, the leader will take his or her place at the water, assisted by one or two other people. Each person will go there and pray to the nature and water spirit, stating out loud what he or she has done or not done that has contributed to this pollution. After this confession, each person places the give-away item on the ground, offering it to the spirit for cleansing. Then they promise out loud to do something specific to maintain this healing. When the last person has gone through, the leader and assistant will convey these gifts to the water and join the rest of the group for a closing prayer.

NATURE AND EARTH

Nature teaches us how to suckle the great Mother Earth. Born out of her continuously fertile womb, the plants and trees are proud to show to us what the natural juice of our mother tastes like and how invigorating and empowering it is to rely on what she gives. Every person with a little spiritual awareness will recognize that Earth is our Mother. They will also find it easy to understand that nature is the most loyal child of Mother Earth. Where this is the case, such as in indigenous cultures, mothers are a true reflection of Mother Earth. They feed their children the same way that the earth feeds nature and us. Their children are constantly tucked to their body, sucking their bare breasts. This is how these children discover their intimate connection to the mother.

Similarly, the earth will never cease to be the mother, and we should never stop being her trusting children. In the context of our relationship with the earth, dependence is good. To deny our dependence on earth is to deny the mother, and to deny the mother is to deny the feminine. A mother whose job is not recognized will develop illness. I wonder if the epidemic of breast cancer is not symptomatic of the denial of the mother in Western culture. I wonder if people's attraction to synthetic food is not a denial of the real mother, the earth who brings forth food. I wonder if the mistreatment of the earth with chemicals, the sexual objectification of things feminine, and the mistreatment of women in general are not symptomatic of a deeply dysfunctional relationship with the mother.

Here is an outline for a ritual aimed at honoring our dependence on the earth. It is called Thanking the Earth and involves bringing gifts to the

Earth Mother in honor of all the nurturing she has given us, regardless of our behavior. First of all, in order for the ritual to receive the stamp of approval of the spirit of nature, it has to take place in the great outdoors. The sacred space is marked with an altar in the form of a mound of earth at its center. This space must also be decorated with yellow candles, plants, stones, flowers, and individual power objects such as animal carvings, ancestral masks, and meaningful pictures, giving it the vitality that speaks directly to the psyche. At ground level is a space especially made to receive the gifts from the participants. They are instructed ahead of time to give serious thought to the kind of gift they can give to the earth spirit to truly show adequate appreciation for the amount of nurturing they have each received in their lives. By the time they show up for the ritual, they already have their gifts ready.

The ritual leader makes the invocation or opening prayer to the earth spirit and nature spirit, setting the intention of the ritual. In it he or she stresses the fact that we are trying to remember how to be grateful to our Mother for standing at our side all these years without expecting anything in return from us. The leader emphasizes the fact that we are most used to taking from her, and now we are trying to learn how to give to her and to each other by replicating her example. The gesture honors the fact that Earth has never faltered in her commitment toward us, and acknowledges our deep dependence on her.

After this, people intone a chant, supported by the beat of a drum. While this is going on, each individual is gently escorted by the ritual leader to the earth altar. There, he or she opens her gift to the earth and expresses the reason why this particular gift is being offered. The gift is presented to everybody, and they shout their enthusiasm. Then it is passed on to the ritual leader, who then officially presents it to the Earth Mother by placing it on the space provided below the altar. Then the giver is escorted back to the crowd, and another person takes his or her turn.

When everyone has gone through this process and returned to the rest of the group, the leader brings the ritual to a close with a prayer of acknowledgment and gratitude. These gifts, which now add a new dimension of aesthetics to the entire shrine, are left there overnight. Usually, perishable gifts such as food are consumed at night by nocturnal animals. These animals are looked at as other children of the earth, invited by her to share in the abundance. The rest of the gifts are randomly redistributed the next day and some are kept as shrine objects for future earth rituals. If what you get is not what you brought, then he or she who brought it becomes your Earth Mother for the year. Thus participants are kept together in an enhanced relationship of mutual attention until the next ritual.

NATURE AND MINERAL

The sight of a tree growing on a rock is always baffling. Seeming to defy natural laws of connection, the tree makes a strong statement about our relationship to the mineral world. There is magic in the way that a seedling can pass through a rock, and we can see here how the earth passes nourishment to the trees and to ourselves through stones.

People feed on the energy coming out of stone, the tiny particles of earth. This is why in my village, regular food from the nature realm of vegetable and animal used to be served in clay pots and calabashes. The food nourishes our bodies while the clay, which contains particles of stone, nourishes the bones of our body by keeping our memory alive. Memory is the food of connection with ourselves and our purposes.

Here is a short ritual rekindling this important aspect of ourselves. It involves handcrafting the things with which to cook the food for our nourishment. First find an area that has clay in it. People will gather there to make pots, cups, dishes, and so forth. If no clay is available, just think of other natural alternatives, and no doubt you will find many possibilities for crafting vessels that connect you to the world of nature. In order to be sacred, the making of these utensils will have to be ritualized. Thus, it must be preceded with an invocation to the nature and mineral spirits. The ritual leader will bring to the attention of these spirits the deep meaning and the purpose of the action to be taken.

Then people are divided into different task forces. One group will make cups, another will make dishes, and so forth. Meanwhile, everyone is singing to the beat of a drum. The ritual is suspended when all the utensils are made and spread in the sun to dry.

The next episode takes place anytime after the drying and firing of these utensils. It involves using these tools to prepare a meal under the open sky, a meal that will be shared among the people who made the utensils at the very place where they made them. During this section, people cooperate in the production of nourishment. They sing during all that time. The cooked meal is then officially presented to the spirit of nature and mineral. After this each person picks another person, and they feed each other. The gesture honors interdependence and community.

NATURE RITUALS AND GIVEAWAYS

The indigenous believe that healing comes in giving more than in getting. So in order to remain energetically healthy, and to reduce the danger of loss, individual as well as collective lives are punctuated by periodic sacrifices, gift giving to Spirit, and countless giveaways. This conviction has given rise to the invention of an enormous number of rituals that are meant to bring something to oneself, and each of these begins by giving something meaningful away. I will briefly touch on some of the most significant of these rituals.

Everyone is interested in some form of prosperity and comfort. To invite more prosperity and comfort into one's life, village people make offerings of food to the nature spirit. They will first spend a great deal of time collecting samples of different types of food. They put these food samples into a clay pot that has never been used. At sunset or sunrise they take the clay pot out into the wood and place it at the foot of a big tree after making a prayer to the nature spirit. In the prayer is usually a mention of the need to have abundance as diverse as the different food samples presented to the nature spirit. The same food can be given instead to someone who is known to be in extreme scarcity.

Another prosperity ritual, which many people prefer because of its social character, is the offering of a feast. At the outset it looks like a party, except that all the food has been first presented to Spirit at a shrine. The giver of the feast never eats any of the food or drink he or she is offering, and everything must be entirely consumed. In the village, it works best when uninvited guests show up at the party. It means that they are Spirit's special guests.

One last common ritual, which is also lots of fun, is the shipping of a miniature cargo of food via a waterway. Here is how it works: People get together and build a small ship. Everyone participates in loading it with symbols of things they would like to have—money, health, love, comfort, and so forth. Money is symbolized by pennies glued onto the ship. Health is symbolized by figurines or medicine objects such as necklaces, amulets, and talismans. Love is represented by hearts and by small red cloths woven like a tie. Comfort is represented by food samples, scented objects, or perfume. The preparation of the ship must be very careful and detailed, with an emphasis on beauty. When it is finished, someone carries it while everyone else follows to a swiftly flowing waterway. There, they pray to the water spirit that it navigate this ship loaded with abundance to its right destination so that the same abundance may return to all a millionfold. People may wonder how to do this without polluting or littering waterways. What is done as a sacred gesture involving Spirit cannot become pollution. From an indigenous point of view Spirit won't let that happen. When salmon give their life away in the water, their death does not litter or pollute the water because it is sacred. So as long as the intention is as clean as can be the waters will replicate the same cleanness. But those who do not see this point of view can just do the ritual at or near to the ocean.

NATURE RITUALS AND MASKS

In the West, when nature is neglected, people often wear masks in order to survive. The mask may be a professional role; it sometimes comes with a suit or a uniform and is a refuge, a place of anonymity. Those who don't wear a mask in this culture risk being hurt, and thus many are driven to find one. The problem is that as people hide behind these masks, they become defined by them and unable to tell the difference between what is natural and what is not. Sometimes they become so profoundly disconnected from their true self that they think that their mask is their true nature.

Nature rituals aimed at unmasking the true self need to begin by addressing the theme of change. The goal is to allow people to relax, which will allow people to let go of their masks and to find out how it feels to be without a mask for a moment. Healing begins when the mask is released from the self, for people can't transform when they are hiding behind them. Talking is often inadequate for helping people drop their masks, and some of the best ways to accomplish this kind of change are through nonverbal forms of ritual, such as dance, and activities that evoke strong emotions. This is what makes tribal communities rely so heavily on rhythm and dance. Rhythm is not entertainment. Rather, it is a tool to shake off the debris of one's unnatural masks. When one is not in rhythm, one becomes depressed. Likewise depression, or being estranged from one's natural magic, shows in being out of rhythm.

An indigenous person can easily identify the mask someone carries by watching that person dance or play a drum. Music and dance are diagnostic tools that bring out of hiding the parts of the body that are masked or that are being subjected to severe control by unnatural forces. The great majority of Westerners carry these constraints around the hips, the upper spinal column, and the face. These parts of the body rarely participate in natural activities in Western cultures. Concerts attract people because the energy of the music challenges the natural self to come out. If people at a concert were to go where their feelings were trying to lead them, they would naturally burst into dance. Instead, more often than not one is expected to refrain from spontaneity and to applaud politely. This is very hard on the spirit. The idea of listening to music or watching performers engage in spontaneous and frenzied rhythm and dance without joining in is indeed unnatural.

Actual mask-making rituals are another way to unmask the self. A group of people can gather, bringing the appropriate materials: gauze strips and plaster of paris or papier-mâché, Vaseline to coat the face (especially the eyebrows) so the mask can be removed easily, paints, cloth, feathers, stones—whatever decorative, natural objects one feels led to bring. The mask-making process is ritualized with an opening invocation, where someone tells Spirit of the group's intent to create masks that will allow transformation. Then people may choose partners. One person applies the Vaseline or oil and then the casting material to the other's face, lets it dry, and removes it. Then they switch.

When the masks are dry, participants decorate them with a view toward bringing to visibility the kind of self that Spirit sees when Spirit looks at us. This requires drawing from the psychic self or the artist. As a result the decorating of the mask is in itself a ritual in which the decorator is almost in a trance state. When everyone has finished decorating their masks they get together to perform the sacred dance of the masks. There is usually nothing prescriptive about the dance because each person moves his or her body in response to the newly discovered spiritual self. In fact it is the spirit in the self who takes possession of the body and moves it.

The cast one makes of one's own face targets the true, hidden self that lies within and that becomes visibly imprinted in the form of the mask. In the many mask-making rituals that I have observed, people have usually succeeded in drawing out their natural self, allowing the mask makers to see and hold their own "other." More often than not, such masks bear a strange resemblance to animals, especially when provided with a final decorative touch.

The element of nature that the mask highlights has a profound power in our lives. If we live a life that denies or ignores our true and natural self, we open ourselves to some of the most painful emotional and psychological problems that a human being can know. The magic of nature can help to break through our defenses and the habits cultivated over a lifetime. It can help us to drop our masks and to reveal to ourselves and others, even for an instant, the nature of the person behind the mask. Meeting for the first time the person who lives behind the mask is usually a powerful and emotional experience, but from the point of view of the indigenous world, that is the person you came to this life to be.

The mask-making ritual, like all rituals of nature, helps people focus on their purpose and reason for being—on the people we would be if we could drop all artifice and pretense and could see our true purpose clearly. Rituals of nature, in the indigenous view, help people transform so that they become more "real"—more respectful of the gifts provided by the natural world, and more attuned to the nature within us, that is, to our own true nature. Healing, by definition, is this process of coming closer to nature—to the nature around us as well as the true nature within.

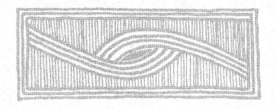

PART FIVE

HEALING IN THE WESTERN WORLD

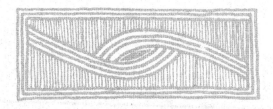

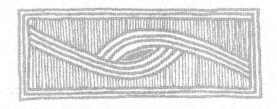

15.

Initiation:
A Response
to Challenges
of the West

Initiatory events are those that mark a man or a
woman's life forever, that pull a person deeper
into life than they would normally choose to go.
Initiatory events are those that define who a
person is, or cause some power to erupt from them,
or strip everything from them until all that
is left is their essential self.
—MICHAEL MEADE,
Men and the Water of Life

We have explored together aspects of healing discovered through finding one's place
in a community, remembering one's true
purpose, and engaging in rituals of fire, wa-

ter, earth, mineral, and nature. In Dagara culture, the experience that puts all these ingredients together is initiation. Rites of initiation are aimed at including the young person in the community and recognizing his or her genius, and moving the youth toward maturity and adult responsibility. Through initiation, a young person gains access to dynamic and purposeful living. While initiation as it takes place in African indigenous culture would not be appropriate in the West, since we are by definition located in a different place and culture, some aspects of initiation would, I believe, speak to particular challenges that Western societies are facing at this time.

Initiation focuses on and is a response to some basic existential questions faced by human beings since the dawn of time. Everyone wonders, Who am I? Where do I come from? What am I here for? and Where am I going?

We have already noted that indigenous people see humans as born with a purpose, a mission they must carry out because it is the reason for their coming to this world. In order to deliver the gift of their mission or purpose, certain conditions must be present, such as the community's recognizing the gift that is being delivered to them.

A spiritual crisis can start as early as birth, when, instead of being welcomed by people, a child meets the silence of technology and cold convention. In this case, a thwarted life purpose surges up during adolescence in the form of impetuousness and insubordination. This behavior is directly linked to the need to enter into a ritual space strong enough to restore the body and the soul's alignment with the purpose of life. It is not coincidental that this time of life brings great physiological changes to a person. These changes are the qualifying signs for rituals of community attention, specifically initiation. If, as in the case of birth, there is no community to respond to the call for a rite of passage, then the youth must feel compelled to respond personally to the fire burning in their belly. This unguided response to a need for an initiatory ritual can have a lethal consequence to the person while testifying to the failure of community.

The youth's attraction to, and fascination with, danger signals the rise in their energetic self of powerful elements that will burn until something is done that will allow a settling catharsis to occur. When this intensity is not responded to with ritual attention, it becomes an incinerating fire directed at the entire society. To the youth, therefore, the production of death and destruction are notices to the village that it must wake up and attend to them or face the consequences of their inattention. Even if the child survives to adulthood and continues to live, looking like a fully integrated man or woman, there is still this undying fire within that continues to burn, defying any chance for contentment and integration. Like a dormant volcano that erupts periodically, such people experience moments of crisis over and over again, prompting them to break through the guardrail of propriety and into some domain of madness frightening to the people familiar with them.

Initiation consists of rituals and ordeals that help young people remember their own purpose and have their unique genius recognized by the community. From birth to puberty, the tribal person is the responsibility of the village; hence the saying that it takes a whole village to raise a child. This collective attention and care prepare the child for the delivery of his or her gift, potential, or skills. Rebirth or rites of passage then mark his/her passage into maturity. Maturity here must be understood as the awakening into one's gift and the investment of self for a good that is greater than self. The mature person therefore is, tribally speaking, the initiated responsible person fully aware of the reasons that brought him/her into this place, committed to carrying out his/her mission with the unconditional support of the village. Initiation thus ritually echoes and completes the passage into life that began at birth.

INITIATION IN THE WEST

Many people in the West dream of a formal indigenous initiation. They have a sense that if they could have this experience, it would put an end to their spiritual yearning by changing their life in dramatic ways. Since my last book, *Of Water and the Spirit,* was published, which deals in large part with initiation, I have been overwhelmed by people requesting that I initiate them, either here in the West, or in my village in Africa. It is as if initiation is a shining pearl that they are driven to acquire. I suspect that their undelivered gift is aching in them and driving them toward this formal ritual.

A Western person who requests initiation from me, however, has misunderstood the connection between initiation and community. Every ordeal of initiation brings the initiate into closer relationship with the community within which the initiate's life purpose will be lived out. I cannot as an initiated person perform initiations for others; initiation does not qualify me for that task, as if it were an academic degree earned in order to train others to attain the same level. Yet constantly I receive requests from people who dream about the day when I will take them to the back country of America and swing open a gateway with a twist of my hand for them to dive into. They envision beholding the Other World crowded with the little people known as *kontombli,* and as a result finding their life problems fixed for good.

But troubles do not befall individuals because of their failure to avoid them. Rather they are milestones of one's journey toward maturity and responsibility. The serious troubles we face in life are nothing other than initiatory experiences. Their aim is to help people better understand what life is, and who we are. They are a necessary ingredient in the removal of whatever stands between us and our essential self. If tribal people reach this stage through formal rites of passage, other people may do the same differently. It is as if there is a natural pull toward challenges and ordeal in the interest of gaining inner strength and living a responsible life. Hardship and ordeal therefore initiate a change from within. One emerges from them with a profound sense of having undergone a radical education. Those who understand this may even come to welcome adversity.

ADVERSITY AS INITIATION

For example, after graduating from college at the age of twenty-two, Robert gets a job, marries, buys a house, and has children. Several years down the road, his trouble begins. His company lays him off, the mortgage is pending, and his wife is not working because she stays home with the children. Tensions mount while the savings drop. Robert cannot get a job easily because there is a recession, and his oldest child gets caught taking drugs at school. Finally, the situation degenerates with loud arguments among the family. The house comes up for foreclosure.

To make things even worse, Robert is informed that he is being sued by his former secretary for rape. She was afraid to come forward while she was still working for him because she feared losing her livelihood, but now that he has left the company, she feels she must speak out. Of course, when the news hits at home, the wife's unhappiness is unlimited. She packs up and leaves, taking the kids, and the house is taken by the bank. Robert is convicted of the rape charge and is sentenced to prison. While in prison, he is forced for the first time in his life really to face himself. So far everything he experiences checks out as initiatory. What is left after he is stripped of everything is himself. This is the only thing he can transform, the germ of his unique genius.

Meanwhile, the economy improves. A good friend is able to help Robert when he is paroled by offering him a good job with his own company. When Robert comes out of prison, his personality is profoundly changed. His vision of life is radically different than it was before. He is determined to be a better father to his children, and he has lost his desire to use women for quick pleasures. In his new job, he applies what he has learned from his ordeal. He does so well that he is eventually promoted to vice president of the company. He begins to work in the area of company employee relations—something he is now an expert at because he has learned from his own struggles. He has also become very alert to human suffering and does not hesitate to tell others who come to him seeking counsel what he himself has experienced.

Robert's experience is an example in every way of a true initiation. It just doesn't have the formality of an indigenous initiation. Such an initiation does not mean that the person is released from suffering forever, but rather that the person is now better equipped to recognize and confront future adversity. Anyone who wants to grow must be prepared to face such problems. It is as if there is something tumultuous about every life path; turmoil is an integral part of it.

Life problems become worse when we expect our growth to be free of thorns and cobbles. Every bump in a person's life is an opportunity to grow and change. Thus, it is not enough simply to regard problems as unfortunate events. One must deliberately attempt to see the potential for growth inside trouble. Being sick, losing a loved one or a job, witnessing a violent death, being overwhelmed by bad news, failing and feeling like a failure: all are opportunities that call us forth, propelling us into the higher grounds of our lives.

It is unlikely that any person in the West, or anywhere in the world, for that matter, has lived thirty years or more without going through some kind of trouble. The social fabric cultivates trouble for us daily. It is as if every day we go out hunting for it, or we are hunted by it; when troubles are resolved, they are not finished. In the path of life new difficulties or challenges, new adversities and bad news lie just ahead. A healthy attitude leads one not to avoid trouble but to move with it. One could conclude that every time a person hurts, something is changing and an initiation is in progress.

Initiation is intimately connected to ordeal. From the point of view of the indigenous, an ordeal stretches the physical self far enough to release something else that brings more awareness, more sense of responsibility and more wisdom. Discipline arises from and is aimed toward acknowledging this: the knowledge that one is going somewhere purposeful in life.

The people I encounter most in my life are usually tired of saying that their lives are fine when, in fact, they are not. They recognize that something initiatory has been going on in their lives that they can no longer deny. For the most part they just want to acknowledge that the end of a marriage is devastating to them, that the loss of their job felt like a stab in their hearts, that the accident they had on the road affected them, that the fact that they had to file for bankruptcy hurt them deeply. They also want to be recognized as survivors, or they want to join a community of survivors.

The wounds left on the psyche by troubles such as the ones mentioned here are signs of initiatory experiences. A wound is an expression of a deep life change in progress. Its completion leaves a scar that reminds its bearer of where he or she has been. A scar seals an event, which prompts a change allowing for a move to another stage. Indigenously defined, a scar is a shrine to the physical or spiritual ordeal undergone by a person. Scars on the body or in the psyche point to some deep changes that occurred as a result of an ordeal.

BRINGING CLOSURE TO INITIATORY EXPERIENCES

Because initiatory experiences are part of every life, the immediate issue for Westerners is perhaps not initiation itself but how one may bring closure to initiatory pain and suffering. People who want to be recognized as survivors are attempting to seal off an initiatory experience so that they can get on with something else, because when suffering is met with recognition, it passes. It is the absence of radical and genuine recognition and acknowledgment that makes suffering grow larger. Initiation and the suffering that accompanies it end when an individual's experiences are acknowledged by others. Radical recognition takes place when a community witnesses and supports the hardship being endured by a person, or the wound he or she suffered.

Among indigenous people, the whole village and sometimes even a series of villages gathers to welcome the initiates back at the end of their ordeals. It is believed that the greater the number of people witnessing and acknowledging the return of the initiates, the better for them, since an ordeal that has not been witnessed and acknowledged is likely to repeat itself.

There is an endless series of unresolved initiations in the modern world due to isolationism and the personalization of trouble. In addition, there is a tendency for many to ostracize people who seek to have their suffering acknowledged. The psyche of a person who seeks recognition as a way to end initiation interprets this ostracism as a sign that the world hasn't noticed, so it sends the message to repeat the experience in hopes that next time someone will take notice.

In the psyche of a person who feels victimized, society owes him or her. Such a person runs a serious risk of acting victimized, looking weak or helpless in a deliberate attempt to attract attention. Thus, people who crave acknowledgment are people who have suffered something deeply within themselves and who know that without such an acknowledgment their suffering is meaningless. In general, people can come to terms with their suffering only if there is a profound translation of their suffering into larger meaning, that is, if suffering serves a greater recognizable good.

Community is key to closing initiation. Without community, people's initiatory experiences are suspended in midair, where they remain ungrounded. The most powerful demonstration of this in the West is perhaps the Vietnam War. This was a collective endeavor in which thousands of individuals were thrown into major initiatory experiences. Is it then surprising that a great number of the homeless are Vietnam veterans? They can't come back because there is no community to welcome them. Their homelessness is brought about by the community's refusal to perceive their experience as initiatory.

The absence of a community to recognize and end suffering is also visible in Westerners' prolonged grief over their parents' inadequacies. On numerous occasions I have seen men and women in their thirties and forties still grieving that their mothers or fathers weren't there for them the way they should have been, that they had "abandoned" them. This crisis in midlife is the result of the person's sense of anonymity and lack of belonging. Indeed, it is important for these people to recognize that their parents were not experts at rearing children. But to hang on to this for many years is symptomatic of a spiritual paralysis. It reveals the isolation of individuals and families from a wider sense of community. When children are raised by a whole village, they do not grow up expecting their biological parents to provide for all their emotional needs.

Lack of a community to bring initiatory ordeals to closure also results in a society of consumers who wander the aisles of a supermarket or browse through a department store in search of fulfillment. When I first came to the West, I would sometimes go to stores just to watch shoppers' behavior. I always emerged bewildered at how perfectly consumerism seemed to console the psyche of so many people. The memory of so many overweight people pushing their overloaded carts up and down the overfull aisles of merchandise, searching for more stuff to load on before proceeding to the checkout counter, continues to amaze me. Every potential purchase is examined in hand with great care, as if it might contain the secret answer. The placement of the item into the shopping cart indicates the buyer's verdict that yes, the answer may be here. Their commitment to addressing the problem that victimizes them by buying more things serves the economy. Meanwhile I can't help but feel that this person needs love, something they won't find on any of the shelves of the supermarket.

Thus, in the West, initiatory experiences rarely come to proper closure. People search for the right thing at the wrong place and blame it on someone else when they find nothing. Attributing blame to someone else can never bring closure to a problem. On the contrary it keeps it alive, near enough to affect us deeply but just too far out of reach for us to solve. Nor can material goods ever fulfill the longing in people's hearts to be recognized for who they truly are and to have both their sufferings and their gifts acknowledged by a community.

In the face of pains that won't go away, or troubles that keep recurring, a common temptation is to embrace them, to become their victim. It is dangerous to accept pain in this way. It is even more dangerous to love suffering and pretend you don't. Time and again I have seen situations in which people looking for help through ritual tried to get rid of their pain. After the initial shock of identifying the deep source of suffering, it turned out that the pain was a person's means of achieving a desirable status, a comfortable place of visibility, bringing them to the center of everybody else's attention.

Most rituals that I do with people in this culture have a direct connection with challenges, pain, and conflict. At the core of these rituals is the commitment to heal a problem that no other medicine can heal. I have had the chance to witness great success in some individuals, but also the frightening realization that certain challenges or pain can survive the onslaught of ritual, either by the participant's pretending that they are gone, or their by becoming obsessed with the attention they naturally receive in the context of a ritual.

I have concluded from this that the problem is not so much the nature of initiation but the absence of a supportive community functioning as a container, recognizing and acknowledging the person's initiatory experience, thereby giving closure to it. And even passing recognition is not enough to terminate an initiation. The person's patterns of life that support the experience of suffering must also be drastically altered. This may include the space in which a person lives, the kind of people he associates with, the type of food he eats, and many other factors that are particular to each individual and situation.

If we begin by accepting the possibility that problems occur because we make them occur—that hardships such as broken relationships, loss of job, financial troubles, and even sickness come because we need them for our own good—then many healing opportunities become available. The question of why I would have invited such a hardship is a good place to begin the journey through initiation. The issue is not how to get out of the hardship as quickly as possible, but how to read the message of change embedded within the hardship. Trouble means that the psyche must move on.

The most common lesson in initiation has to do with control, with holding on to the way things are and resisting change. Whether we understand what the trouble is telling us or not, it is imperative to bring the trouble into ritual. What follows, in ritual, should inspire the mind to change its approach to crisis.

THE THREE STAGES OF INITIATION

It is not too hard for an indigenous eye to notice that initiations are taking place at all times and in every town and city in the West. At every moment, many people are going through some form of initiatory experience. This means that many people are going through suffering they would rather avoid. For purposes of dealing with initiatory experiences, whether in the context of formal rituals, or as they are encountered in our daily life, it can be useful to understand them as a three-stage process.

In the early stage, the trouble or ordeal has just started. For example, Susan has worked for a company for many years. She never thought of, nor ever concerned herself with, the possibility of being laid off until she received a pink slip. Suddenly, her uneventful life becomes loaded with stormy potentials. The journey into the unknown has just begun. Similarly Steve, a healthy strong man, never thought very much about illness beyond minor flu and colds until he was told that he was HIV positive. In another case, a friend of mine came crashing onto the sofa of my office announcing between sobs that his wife just left him. These are the visible manifestations of powerful initiatory beginnings. They come as a shock. These kinds of events one would rather not be involved with.

The middle stage is a period of extreme disruption. It is a place of deep chaos where everything seems to be plotting against oneself. It is as if at every corner hides some new trick to complicate further what is already almost unbearably bad. People caught in it are on the high seas of their initiatory journey. They can't see the shore in either direction. They feel alone, lost, resentful that bad fortune has chosen them. For example, when a romantic relationship grows sour, everything one tries in the interest of resolving the crisis feels like fuel poured onto fire, yet it is clear that action must be taken to rescue the situation.

With the end stage comes, at last, a view of the shore. More often than not the shore is as hard to reach as the middle stage is to endure. Sometimes one reaches the shore and finds it impossible to locate a safe harbor. The end is achieved through countless attempts to dock, for example in the relationship that ends with separation but where one partner cannot let go of the other. Haunted by the specter of the lost love, it feels as if nothing in the world will make a proper closure possible. The ongoing patterns that result are unresolved initiations.

Wherever one fits in these three stages of initiatory journeys, the key is to escape isolation. That is, it is important not to approach the process as a private secret one, but to seek out others who may be on the same road in order to travel the path with them. Again, we're talking here about community. Pain is frightened when too many people are involved, when too many people are talking about it and examining it. Pain likes to be kept in silence, nurtured in the darkroom of the psyche. That's when it sets out its roots and begins to grow healthy and vigorous. If suffering is our guest, and it flourishes and grows, this is because we are an excellent host. To be a good host means to provide VIP treatment, giving our suffering excessive and unnecessary attention, which can degenerate into a certain love of suffering. This is what happens when people make themselves into the story of their suffering. So pain decides to move into the psyche, and if it is well treated, it invites every friend and relative to come and join.

A RITUAL FOR RECOGNIZING INITIATIONS

The pain of initiation is best managed through ritual. Here is an example: People gather and divide into groups based on their initiatory stage, early, middle, or final. Each group selects a spokesperson. Each group builds an altar or a shrine on which participants place a sacred object, a power object. The sum of the power objects on each altar represents the Spirit community in direct connection with the human community formed by the group. In a semicircle formation facing the altar, the group can sing songs as a way to open the space to the palpable presence of Spirit. The group leader can then make a general prayer to the community of gods and goddesses with a stress on the purpose of the gathering. One person then steps forward, sits before the group facing the altar, and communicates to Spirit in prayer form the nature of the initiatory experience he or she is going through. Meanwhile, the rest of the group plays the role of witness, carefully listening to what is being said.

At the end of each painful disclosure, the group leader makes an intercessory prayer on behalf of the group member, stressing the fact that he or she needs the help of Spirit to complete the initiation properly, and must come back and join his people in order to carry out his life mission. The prayer would run something like this: "O Spirit, you understand more than anyone else the meaning of what we just heard. Please stand on the side of our brother/sister. Walk him/her through the darkness of this path. Bring him/her home to us. Our village needs the beauty of his/her heart. . . ." Every sentence of the intercession prayer is spoken slowly and deliberately, then repeated by the rest of the group so that there is a sense of community assisting the individual. At the end of the prayer, the person in the center of the group stands up, then turns around to face each member of the group. The group intones a chant while, one by one, people walk to the individual, give a welcome embrace, and utter a welcome word in that person's ear.

The effect of this ritual on the recipient can be tremendous. First of all, the feeling is overwhelming. All of a sudden, pain and confusion dissipate as a sense of belonging creeps in. The sense of this being an individual problem goes away and is replaced by the powerful presence of collectivity. The individual is thereby equipped with what it takes to solve the puzzle of his ordeal. In order for this to work, each participant must be very sincere. Note also that this ritual is designed for adults who are in the depths of one form of trouble or another.

INITIATION AND WESTERN YOUTH

It is clear that young people become painfully aware of the lack of community support as they grow up. Their disdain and mistrust of adults is an expression of their disappointment that society doesn't allow them to embrace life the way they see it. They see the sacred dimension of life, they smell the presence of the Other World. It is fearsome yet attractive. They require community support in order to embrace the initiatory ordeals that will lead them to the beauty they naturally seek and to the gift they have. Street gangs have evolved as a direct response to the feeling of ostracism by the community. They are an expression of what society does not want to look at. They provide an alternate initiatory circle to their members, no matter how dangerous and displaced they may be.

We have in the West a situation that is extremely destructive to youth. This situation looks as though it could benefit from a little indigenous wisdom such as initiation and the need for community to raise a child. The perplexity of society in the face of gangs and violence, or the prison approach to it, suggests that deep down modern people are still at a loss as to how to cure this basic human crisis.

What would a formal initiation for youth in the modern world look like? This is a question I have been asked many times and to which I have no definite answer. What follows is what I might try if I were to lead young people into an initiatory experience. The first step would be to separate the geography of community and the geography of initiation. In this case, nature seems to be the most desirable space for initiation since the experience is much more connected to nature than to the urban world. The youth must be taken into a natural space and allowed to spend sufficient time there to gain an awareness of its inhabitants, its trees, animals, stones, and spirits. The general content of this process, which must be given sufficient time, would include periods of isolation with the elements of nature, and periods of coming together with other youth for communal handling of an ordeal. The magic would arise from the youth's discovery of his own worth and a sense of purpose in his life.

A more detailed form of this initiation might begin with some form of induction, which in my village might be the ritual removal of hair and the decoration of the head with paint obtained from the bark of a tree. People involved with leading such an initiation must conceive of a way to change the physical appearance of the initiates so that the psyche can adjust to what is supposed to happen thereafter. We believe that painting patterns on the body, for example, alters the body's energy, and it is easily achievable, as is shaving the head.

The next thing is to arrange a number of ordeals for the initiate to pass through. These ordeals must be sensitive to the geography and the already existing customs. Tribal initiation offers five different types of ordeal that are adjusted to fit the needs of particular circumstances. The ordeals can follow the pattern of five elements outlined already. One is the fire ordeal. Its significance involves connecting with the ancestors, with one's deep past. The question here is how can fire be used in a radical ritual context to incinerate an unwanted self, thereby liberating the new self? Certainly the heat of fire must be experienced and its intensity must match the intensity of youth. If this ritual involves a large fire in which initiates burn something of themselves, the experience of heat sustained in the interest of cleansing will achieve the purpose wanted.

Next is the water ordeal. Water is seen as the peacemaker and the reconciler. The challenge here is how to experience water in ways shocking enough to constitute a memorable ordeal. This might include submerging or pouring over, or even diving into water in search of something hidden. The exact choreography of this stage is solely the responsibility of the initiators who would be familiar with the purposes and participants of the ritual.

The earth ordeal responds to the youth's need to be in touch with themselves and with the ground. Here the issue is how initiates can be reintroduced to the power of the earth to give and to renew life. How can the earth be reunderstood as an earth womb large enough to swallow an initiate long enough for a shift to occur in the person? A few hours' burial in the earth can work. The feeling of being in the earth is radically transforming.

The mineral ordeal usually takes the form of a journey to find one's stone amidst a vast field of stones. One purpose of this is that the stone becomes the token of one's initiation, constantly reminding the initiate of what has happened in their life.

The nature ordeal must involve a journey into nature, or an experience with nature that results in deep transformation. It could be as simple as spending the whole day with a single tree, meditating with it, looking at it, talking to it. Young people can sometimes hear the sound of plants. We must trust them to listen and to collect information about them from the trees themselves. This exercise can take place either during the day or at night.

Each one of these ordeals must be given ample time to evolve. A twenty-four-hour period that begins with a detailed presentation and preparation, followed by the five ordeals, and concluding with some kind of recovery stage should be quite successful. This gives time for the initiates to process what they have experienced. Meanwhile, the initiators can fine-tune their strategies through close observation of how initiates respond to the entire process.

Meanwhile, at home, there must be some kind of preparation for the return of the initiates. The reception of initiation participants must be as warm and sincere as possible, making the youth realize how important it is to be part of the community. Warm welcomes have positive effects on the human psyche. They increase your sense of belonging and help you feel better. It is important for someone who has undergone an ordeal to know that after all they are not alone. Above all, it is transforming to be made to feel like a hero. This feeling has the effect of sealing the individual's commitment to whatever serves the greatest common good.

When planning rituals of initiation for young people, it is important to keep in mind that it takes someone other than parents to initiate children.

In no indigenous community are parents directly involved with the initiation of their children. This is because it is not the role of a parent to do such a thing. In initiation, as in other areas of child raising, adults other than parents are needed so that children can receive all the facets of love and support and guidance that they require. Children will learn best how to see their problems as initiatory with the help of mentors and elders. If the parents have held the space for the children to grow, and have introduced other adults into their children's lives, these mentors and elders will not be missing when needed.

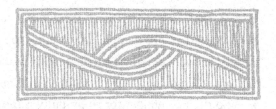

16.

Maintaining Community Through Ritual

Every Westerner who visits my village leaves with
one thing, and that is the experience of the
intensity of human connection and attention.
It is not the magic, the ritual or the ceremonies
that are done, but an awareness of the intensity
of human connection that they take away.
This is what makes them long to return again,
because that is what they don't get here.

What would it be like if that intensity of human
connection could be found here, in addition to
all of the material wealth that is available?
If the human wealth could match the material
wealth, what would happen? Heaven could
be created, right here.

—MALIDOMA SOMÉ

In my workshops and seminars throughout North America and Europe, I have found that what people most want is to satisfy their hunger for community, to dwell in radical ritual for their healing, to bring to a happy conclusion their strong desire for belonging, and to understand and work with Spirit. The hunger for community is the most difficult subject to address, because it arises within a society that is established against a village type of community, and because participation in a community is a precondition for true ritual healing, for a sense of belonging that satisfies, and for a rewarding understanding of Spirit. Among the most frequent questions asked by seminar and workshop participants are questions about how to form communities that work. People talk of "intentional communities" they once belonged to but that brought them more harm than before, and they wonder why community is so much needed and yet so hard to achieve.

It is hard for me to witness the sometimes irresistible desire for community when I realize how unable I am to supply clear definitive answers that can be readily applied. I feel the pain of those who want to leave behind their present state of disconnection, and I deeply want to do something about it. But whatever I do feels as though it is not enough. Time and again I have felt like an indigenous Moses assigned the task of leading a special people out of the grip of some demonic hands, across the Red Sea of their despair, and into the land of spiritual milk and honey.

Sometimes, after a weekend or a five-day event where we all have immersed ourselves in deep rituals, people reach the end feeling even greater worries. Their concern borders on panic. They ask, "How do we keep the intensity we have experienced here while out there?" They fear that the deep sense of community, of connection, that they experience in the protected quiet of a camp will evaporate shortly after they reintegrate into the world.

The solution, perhaps, lies elsewhere than in one man or woman showing everyone else the way out. That model is too messianic. The better answer comes from within. But in order for the answer to emerge from within people, they will need some model that fuels their imagination and creativity. In other words, I do not have all the answers to the problems the West is facing, but I know that, offered an alternative model, Western people can take it and adapt it to their own situation. The following is an attempt to sow some seeds for creative men and women eager to contribute to community. It is not and should not be a ready-made answer to a perennial problem.

FINDING COMMUNITY IN THE WEST

Where is community found in the West? To the extent that humans live better in community, there has to be community in the West in one form or another, otherwise Western society would cease to exist. The real question, and the challenge, is whether the communities that do exist have the interest and the adaptability to absorb the work of ritual as a way of addressing conflict and as a way of addressing the many social problems that require some healing energy but which seem so insoluble for now. Communities take many forms in Western culture, and most of them are struggling for their very survival. The struggle indicates that they need to change somehow so they can protect the individuals within them more effectively, holding them with greater love and respect. The hope for such change to occur comes from the fact that individuals in the West are deeply yearning for a more genuine kind of community that can offer a deeper sense of belonging.

Clearly the form that community assumes in the West is not the same as an indigenous form of community. Many groups invite belonging in modern society, and any context that has a movement toward belonging has the potential for becoming community. Religious and spiritual groups, neighborhood organizations, groups of co-workers, and all of the countless organizations that bring people together are all attempts at forming some type of community. But religious and spiritual groups often become more interested in maintaining their own structure than in embracing the individuality of each of their members. Societies and or-

ganizations put more energy into maintaining their public image or pre-
serving their by-laws and the positions of those in power than in listening
and adapting to what each individual needs. Community organizations
become more interested in what the front of your house looks like than in
what is going on with the people inside of the house.

People are looking for a place where their individuality will be honored, where their personal gifts can be freely made available to serve the
greater good. From this strong desire to belong, people form groups, only
to find that belonging involves maintaining some sort of uniformity; and
so to satisfy their strong craving to be included, people sacrifice their individuality, becoming casualties of their own desire for belonging. This is
seen in its extreme form in the mass popular culture of the West, which di-
lutes the individual tremendously until his or her identity is done away
with, replaced by a clonelike uniformity. Community will always fail, and
fail those it is supposed to serve, when belonging takes place through
maintaining uniformity. I think that the need for uniformity is prompted
by the mystery of the other. If people were not mysteries to one another—if every individual were known in-depth in the way we've described earlier—there would be little or no attraction to uniformity.

The desire for community that truly fulfills the needs felt by every individual is not diluted in the West, even though people's expectations to
be seen for who they are, to be appreciated, and to be wanted are not being met in modern culture. There are lessons in the ways that indigenous
communities unite and sustain themselves that are relevant and adaptable
in the West. In indigenous cultures, people relate to one another in terms
of what each brings to the village, not in terms of how each one appears.
A chief is only a keeper of a particular power that people respect deeply.
To separate the person behind the role from the role as chief, a yearly ritual is organized in which the chief must cook food and serve it to
everybody all by himself. So, in a sense, a chief is not a chief; a chief is a
person who happens to bring a particular set of gifts to the community.

This is why people of great material deprivation, the very thing that the West is trying to avoid, find themselves loaded with the power to give more than those who have great material wealth. The best they can give, all that they can give, is themselves. Every Westerner who visits my village leaves with one thing, and that is the experience of the intensity of human connection and attention. It is not the magic, the ritual, or the ceremonies that are done. It is not the lurking presence of envy, greed, anger, for in these respects the tribal person is not too unlike the Western person. But an awareness of the intensity of human connection is what visitors take away. This is what makes them long to return again, because that is what they don't get here in the West.

What would it be like if that intensity of human connection could be found here, in addition to all of the material wealth that is available? If the human wealth could match the material wealth, what would happen? Heaven could be created, right here.

ENHANCING COMMUNITIES THROUGH RITUAL

As we have seen throughout this book, ritual is the cement that bonds the individual to the greater community in the Dagara culture. Ritual takes us to an unfamiliar place. Over there, we momentarily lose our mundane sense of orientation and familiarity. This is why for ritual to succeed, each individual is asked to give up their desire to control or to be in control. The group agrees that in order to heal the problems and conflicts that plague its members, everybody has to turn to Spirit.

The space of Spirit is not familiar to everyone. This unfamiliarity can appear frightening, but when a part of you becomes willing to proceed with a ritual, you find that the reward is worth the momentary loss of control. You enter a space where you are allowed to feel, allowed to move, allowed to cry, allowed to feel true compassion for the people you are with. The value that you have in ritual space comes from your personal gifts and from the knowledge that you must depend on the personal gifts of others for your own needs to be met. This profound sense of recognition creates a powerful and lasting bond among people, because they feel seen and heard.

To bring ritual to the communities that already exist in the West in a manner that will emphasize the true identity of community requires, first, that we redefine ritual. The images and the notions of ritual that are predominant in the West have little to recommend them. We must therefore redefine ritual in such a way that it appeals even to those who have been turned off or alienated by the usual ones. Ritual is what brings community together and what truly heals the individual.

Through the energy of emotion, the practice of ritual fosters a splendid openness of people toward one another and a sense of intimate connection with the whole group and with nature. The modern world, as we have seen, inhibits the expression of people's true nature, so ritual will help awaken people's hidden capabilities. Even indigenous people, who live in close proximity to the natural world, still require the practice of ritual in order to maintain a healed self and a sense of connection to the natural world. Those who are detached from nature, as are modern people, therefore not only will have to practice ritual, they also will have to live inside a ritual space in order first to awaken that natural self and then to maintain it.

Doing a ritual once is not sufficient to awaken gifts that have lain dormant in a person for a lifetime, for it is only by inserting the self in the repeated practice of ritual that one gives these gifts the room to emerge. Until this dormancy is awakened, the person remains incomplete, unavailable, and incapable of fully blossoming. Ritual, in the context of awakening the dormant and unexpressed parts of a person, is aimed directly at the individual's psyche; it is a language of invocation, inviting the inner self to come out. For the inner self to show itself in the individual, it must be invoked over and over and over until it does.

When people who are committed to a group, be it their church, their club, or any other group, become aware that something inside themselves still is not being called forth in their group, a first step is to call on the elements of nature. The group gathers together to find out what the elements of nature can offer that will contribute to a further awakening. A natural place to begin is with the element earth, since for the Dagara people it is Earth that provides us with a sense of nourishment, empowerment, and recognition. It is precisely these qualities that can deepen the sense of community in a group, for the feeling of loving affinity that we yearn for grows out of the experience of giving and receiving undivided attention within a group. This loving recognition provides true comfort.

A group of people who decide to bring the element earth into their midst might go out onto a hill somewhere and collect dirt and put it right in the center of the place where they meet. They would decorate it in any way that feels appropriate, thus creating a shrine to the earth. The members of the group could acknowledge that we are all walking on the earth, it is nourishing us, so we can draw from its example and try to replicate that sense of nourishing, empowering, and acknowledgment among ourselves.

The group would begin by identifying those members who are naturally serving, nurturing, and caring, who are then put in charge of the empowerment of each person so that everyone feels attended to and nourished. The ritual might begin with a prayer to the Earth Mother, saying, "Hey, Mother, listen to us. We have been missing the sense that we are valued and paid attention to. We have not always felt we were being fed with what we needed. We have been missing the sense of touch that you can give us. Maybe this is because we have not been listening to you and following your example, so here and now we are going to try to replicate for each other what you do for us. We will allow our feet to touch you when we walk. We will draw with great gratitude from the food that comes from your bosom to feed ourselves, and each of us recognizes that we do not always pass on to each other the abundance that you so freely give us. We are going to try here to reproduce you as best we can in our gathering today."

After this general prayer, a song would be in order of praise to the earth, to the archetypal Mother and caretaker, to whatever the earth symbolizes for the group. The people who have volunteered to serve and act like the earth then take a position around the mound of dirt that has been decorated. One by one, the people would come to the earth shrine and lie down on the dirt and allow themselves to be touched, to be talked to, to be made to feel as though they were the most important person in the world. Each individual is then carried or led back to the larger group, where with great joy they are introduced with the announcement, "Open your hearts and welcome this person, for they have come back to you again!" The person is embraced, welcomed, and recognized by the gathered village.

After giving only ten or twenty minutes of such attention to each member, you will find that you are opening up a totally different dynamic in the group. This kind of activity can be welcomed by everyone without objection, because it is given by the very people who want to experience a sense of community, and that is what makes it work. The members of the group become their own experts, taking the steps that are necessary to make their group feel a lot more genuine to them, with a greater sense of belonging for everyone. The dramatic effect that a group can experience from even such a simple exercise can demonstrate to each person that they have something to give in their ability to show love and attention with a touch, a feeling, a word that is very simple yet extremely powerful and healing. When this awareness is awakened in people, they are changed forever. Every time I have gone through a ritual similar to this with a group of people, I have seen them strive to give one another more than they ever intended to give at the start, deliberately trying to maintain the atmosphere of genuine attention to one another.

A ritual such as this is not voodoo. There is no priest, magician, or sorcerer involved or required. It involves only touch, which is something we are all able to do, and saying nice words, which means simply giving attention. Carrying someone back to the larger group after they have been touched by the earth, saying simply, "Here is this person that you know, welcome them with your hearts," is quite simple but far from simpleminded. It involves recognizing that a person, no matter how familiar they are to us, needs to be taken out of the familiar and reintroduced to everyone as though that person had just arrived. In that moment each person's esteem for themselves and for others in the group is reset. Nature is the textbook for this exercise. It tells us how much we are cared for by the earth and shows us how we can better relate to and support one another.

The ritual described above cements the bond between the individuals in a community, providing the group with a sense of its own identity. In a very small group, this ritual can be accomplished quite simply and easily. But in a larger group of, say, one hundred people—a group the size of a small indigenous village—a significant investment of time and energy needs to be made. The group might set aside an Earth Week, with several hours spent each day in ritual in order to provide the twenty to thirty minutes of close attention required for each person. When the last person has gone through this process, this community is cemented and bound together for the next year to come.

RITUAL AND DIVERSITY

The attention that each person receives in ritual becomes a permission to let loose the innate gifts that the person has, including the particular manner in which that person knows how to provide their gifts. The gifts you have to give and the manner in which you make your gifts available to the people around you translates into and secures an identity that is particular to you.

Because you have been given love, attention, and care, you don't feel threatened or uneasy about the particular way you choose to serve your community, you just do it. Others accept and love you and do not want to censure anything that you might wish to offer. Indigenous people have been caring for one another in this way for a long time. When an outsider looks at indigenous culture and sees the devotion to community held by its individuals, it looks to them as if the individual self has been annihilated. For the person inside such a community, however, the sense of respect and value for one's own original and unique identity is tremendous, and it results in the desire to remain in the community because that is where your genuine identity is guaranteed the right to blossom fully.

Any community that begins with a mission statement and a set of by-laws, any group that believes that it has an identity and purpose before it has ever even asked anyone to join, will fall short of serving the true needs of each of its individuals. Any group that demands that its members follow a preexisting set of rules and by-laws can therefore never be a true community. The character of any true community can be seen only when each of its members has been awakened fully and allowed to reveal his or her innate gifts and genuine self. The sum of all of these unique identities then becomes the character and identity of the community. A healthy community not only supports diversity, it requires diversity.

Within the individuals in a community are all of the gifts and skills necessary to sustain that community. When these gifts are not known or are not available, then communities often turn to creating hierarchies to try to maintain themselves, with everyone coming to the minister, or the mayor, or the leader to try to get what they need. Someone is defined as a leader or is placed in a special position of power, with the assumption that that person is the intermediary between the community and the rest of the world. The sense of community should develop in such a way that the responsibility involves everybody. In the language of the Dagara, everyone is a gatekeeper; everyone has the responsibility to hold open the gate of his or her particular gift on behalf of the whole community.

The roles that people fill to meet the needs that arise in an indigenous community are not rigidly defined; people do not in general have fixed functions. When you find you need something from someone else, you do not travel around until you find the one person with the expertise you require. Rather, it is indigenous people's experience that a need draws to itself that which is needed to fulfill it. Once a need is clearly articulated and understood, indigenous people would say that the need highlights the person who will provide for that need. This is seen as a type of causality, that when a need expresses itself, the means to satisfy that need becomes manifest. In this way, everyone's gifts are used in the community, and the presence of the community enhances and makes possible the expression of individual, diverse gifts.

For example, I recall when I returned home to my village at age twenty after all those years suffered in colonial French schools. I was a time bomb ready to explode. I was angry and resentful toward my parents for conspiring with the colonial power, in the form of the local French Jesuit priest, to let me be taken from the village as a child. But my fiery emotion was a strong request for a mentor and for initiation. I did not have to go out looking for a mentor, nor did I have to search for an initiatory experience. Both came in response to the intensity of my desire. My need drew forth the man who became my mentor. In a similar way, the needs of the youth of my village for guidance upon entering adulthood had led the practices of initiation to be developed, and through the process of initiation my fires were quenched and the guidance I needed was provided.

HEALING CONFLICT THROUGH RITUAL

Modern society feels stuck in its inability to deal with conflict. In the West people usually translate the problem into some type of either/or duality, where someone is right and someone is wrong, someone is a winner and someone a loser. Conflict becomes an opportunity for instant polarization. Wherever polarity exists, there is a state of competitiveness that usually does not serve to meet the needs in a community, since it tends to separate rather than unite. Polarity and the competitive climate it produces encourage concealment, the real omission of truth, and sometimes even conniving and conspiring. Conflict that degenerates into polarity is seldom resolved and breeds problems that become viruses in the society that usually incubate into bigger conflicts.

Indigenous societies concede the existence of conflict but view it as something of importance and of interest to the community. The conflict is some sort of message directed to the entire community but expressed through the individuals embroiled in the conflict. Interpersonal conflict is therefore not really interpersonal to the indigenous; all conflict is community conflict. The message for the community that lies behind the friction two people are experiencing must be assimilated and resolved successfully to serve the greater good of the community.

Besides the difference between the "I" and the "you" that triggered the strong energy that we call conflict, there is another dynamic, another force—the indigenous would say a spirit—that is trying to communicate something to the two of us and to everybody else. This is why, when conflict arises between two people in the village, the first place where that conflict is handled is in the sacred space of ritual. Ritual provides a way of getting past the simple differences that are polarizing a relationship so that the conflict can become an opportunity for those in the relationship to come closer together. Conflict becomes an occasion for people to enter into a ritual intimacy.

That there is a value to the community to be found in the interpersonal friction that arises among people has been a hard concept for many of the Western groups that I have worked with. It is strange how Westerners get uncomfortable about face-to-face confrontation. Perhaps this is why they prefer to be isolated from each other. When viewed in an indigenous fashion—as something natural and constructive—friction is much healthier than anonymity. Western dislike of open confrontation actually invites deeper conflict. Fear of the frictional side of relationships has led to a harsh individualism that many find very hard to bear.

It is true that no one should look forward to friction because it was not designed with sweetness in it, but one must be able to accept friction when it must happen for the benefit of the community. Real friction is aimed at deepening the communal sense. I have seen many examples in the West where a group trusted each other enough to take an issue into the space of ritual that looked, on the surface, like some sort of very personal disagreement between two of its members. In the invocation, Spirit is asked to bring the light of truth, clarity, and understanding about the message contained in the misery between the two people. The outcome of such a ritual cannot be predicted, but in the end, the expression of heartfelt emotion has usually touched and involved everyone. The issue between the two people who were initially in conflict may not look totally resolved, but the energy of the friction is usually much softer, and the connection between their problem and the rest of the community looks much clearer.

Consider the conflicts that occur between a husband and a wife. When the two experience a conflict, the question to be asked is, is this simply friction between two people who live closely together, or does it concern the way in which their relationship and intimacy need to be permitted to grow? If simple discussion does not resolve the differences, then the conflict is taken into a ritual. The parties involved are taking their issues not to the ears of a human tribunal but to the ears of the ancestors and spirits, who listen to those words spoken in a sacred space. This approach to conflict is not about making someone right and someone wrong in order to be fair. We all know that hurt feelings are not healed because someone is right. In relationships, hurt is painful, whether the hurt is right or wrong.

The ritual work begins with each partner offering their version of the story of the conflict to a sacred source, speaking openly and candidly of their experience. Each person says, "This is how it feels to me!" Others who are present are a silent audience, listening carefully for clues in the stories that will point to a need for additional ritual work to resolve the problem ultimately for the couple and the village. For example, a husband and wife have run into conflict over responsibility for the family's resources. They tell their stories in a sacred space, each lamenting about how the other's irresponsibility has damaged the family. The appointed listeners hear that the problem began many years before, when scarcity became an issue throughout the region. The wife had been brought up to share everything with everybody. She cannot understand why abundance must be kept to oneself when others are suffering, so she has been giving away food liberally. The husband, who is more up to date, does not want to share the fruit of his sweat. He sees his wife as wasteful. To heal the earlier wound, the listeners recommend a ritual cleansing. The partners discover that their conflict is resolved when the earlier problem is addressed in a separate ritual.

Another couple comes to the sacred space, experiencing conflict over the slow cooling off of their relationship. They speak about how the coldness of the other makes them feel. This time the listeners do not hear of some deeper problem affecting the marriage or the village. In their case, as is often true, the simple process of telling their stories in a sacred space allows all the feelings of conflict to melt away.

The next step of the process is a ritual involving the entire village. This step is required even when the storytelling alone managed to diffuse all heat and friction. Others in the village become the mouth speaking on each partner's behalf, explaining what is happening. Each speaker emphasizes how important each of the partners is to the greater good of the village. There is no discussion about who is right or wrong. This portion of the ritual is not dissimilar to the earth ritual described at the beginning of this chapter, in that members of the community are affirming the worth of each person. People in conflict need to have their own importance reaffirmed by others, since the parties in conflict cannot do this for each other. The community is the one capable of giving the undivided attention that can reempower people. When the parties to the conflict are brought back together, they now have the strength that allows them to realize how much the energy of the conflict they felt went beyond themselves. The problems of two people have been collectivized.

People bound by marriage are sure, at some point, to get on each other's nerves. It is natural, for tight connection breeds friction. This is so true that, in my village and some other villages in Africa, every five days couples must enter into a ritual space to renew their relationship for another five days. Here is how it takes place.

Shortly before sunrise, the man and woman come together in a place open to the sky. They each bring water and ash. Water symbolizes peace and life. Ash symbolizes protection. The ash is used to draw either a circle to contain the couple or as a straight line between the two parties, who position themselves facing away from each other. Two bowls of water are kept on the side for the closure of the ritual. Each one fills their mouth with water and turns their back toward the other. After a while, in deadly silence, they spit the water out of their mouths, turn toward each other, and begin screaming at each other madly. There is no physical violence involved, but if you were to listen to the intensity coming out of each mouth, you would think that these people never cared for each other at all, that they had been mortal enemies forever.

The point is not to stop and listen to what the other is saying but to scream out every upsetting thing that the other did in the last five days. The ritual doesn't last very long, perhaps because of its vicious intensity. While still screaming at each other, one of them leans down and grabs their bowl of water and the other follows suit. At almost the same time, they drench each other with the water, thereby bringing the ritual to an end. The catharsis is immediately felt as tears come and grief flows. The general feeling before and during the ritual is uncomfortable, but the sense of release afterward is cathartic. This suggests that even healthy relationships need a ritual, because ritual provides a container for friction within the sacred.

There are dire consequences in an indigenous society when problems that are intended for a collective solution are held personally and privately. When Christianity came into tribal communities, it taught people to try to deal with their problems privately, at great cost to village stability. A villager joins the new creed. He is asked to destroy every shrine and fetish in his house to embrace Christ fully and be at peace. After doing so, illness hits one of the members of his family. He takes the issue to the priest, who provides medication and recommends prayers. Everyone else in the village knows that the problem is a warning because Spirit is angry. But to the new convert, this problem is his problem, and God will take care of it. Soon enough, his family member dies.

Shortly after the funeral, he himself falls sick. The priest tells him it is just a case of bad flu, gives him medication, and tells him to pray. The village says the ancestors are getting angrier. Members of the family are beginning to lose their patience, while others think some miracle may still happen. A village healer warns him that unless a public ritual is done on his behalf, he will surely die. In a moment of panic, he tells of his parting with the ancestors and agrees that the ritual be done. Though he heals, he must still carry the remorse over the death of one of his family members. This may sound like a hypothetical case, but it took place in my own family. My father bears the scars of grief over lost family members after he converted to Christianity. He was able to heal after returning to the ancestral rituals, but his loss was severe.

When an individual nurtures a problem, usually a problem in the family that has not been made public, that person carries the family conflict out into the community, where she or he is likely to continue the conflict with others. To be vulnerable to attack by someone in this way is symptomatic of your also carrying some problem personally that needs to be brought to the community and collectivized. Real and lasting damage takes place when something that is supposed to happen in a sacred place has been brought instead into the profane openness of daily life.

All of this would not make sense if I were not convinced that Western people can adapt these practices even in the face of all their contrary training and habits. But the exact way to accomplish this is up to them. The great gift that every Westerner has is creative imagination. This is all it takes to adapt practices that speak to their needs.

From an indigenous perspective, the way Western societies approach accountability takes a painful toll on the individual. Indeed, accountability can relate to pride in one's work, and it can serve as a guardrail in one's relationships. But accountability can also produce other, unwanted, results. If accountability means being punished for what you did wrong or being blamed for a mistake, then accountability is likely to freeze the human fire and have a destructive impact on the individual's connection with community. People fearing the devastating consequences of accountability for the rest of their lives can be drawn to self-destruction or to very hostile actions against their community.

The indigenous alternative offers an opportunity. In it accountability means something like a deepening of the connection with the thing or the person you wronged. If you cause harm to someone, accountability means doing something that brings you close to the person on a regular basis for as long as you live. This is why serious, close relationships can often be traced back to a devastating start.

I am deliberately trying to stress here the necessity of ritualizing conflict. It is acceptable and proper for individuals to have conflicts with others, as long as their arguments are voiced within a space that is considered sacred. This space in village culture is maintained by an elder who mediates. It seems as if it would help people in Western culture who are eager to resolve conflicts first to appreciate the importance of the elder and the sacred. It often appears to me that the failure to resolve personal conflicts, family conflicts, conflict on the job, and so forth, comes from thinking that one's own creative resources can substitute for the guidance of the elder and the sacred. A wife who complains to her husband that he is neglecting his children would gain a better hearing from her husband in a context that is sacred. The sacred and the elder protect both parties by placing around them a ring of respect. It is my sense that the fear of open conflict in the West can be traced to the latent longing for ritual space and for the elder.

For a community to appreciate the collective meaning behind the maladies of any of its individuals requires an open mind in the truest sense. Similarly, for a community to act responsibly based on the messages that are presented to it in this way by Spirit requires a level of integrity and cohesiveness within the community that is not easily attained. A community's stage in its own development determines its ability to handle relationship problems. The more open to Spirit the members of the community are and the more attentive to the emotional needs of each individual member, the better able the community will be to address the conflicts that will inevitably surface. Again, it would be naive for me to think that community practices relevant to an indigenous village can easily be transplanted to a Western context, but what is indeed possible is a deepened commitment to fostering the unique genius of each individual and an increased willingness to listen for Spirit's guidance.

COMMUNAL RITES OF PASSAGE

The project of creating and maintaining community is a deeply involving one. Even after a ritual such as the earth ritual described above, during which people open up so much in an emotional outpouring that brings greater intimacy among the people, you have to continue doing rituals in order to maintain that kind of energy. Otherwise people go back home and begin again to personalize their problems. This will translate in the group dynamics into some people becoming vulnerable to being picked on or to treating others poorly. Nothing perfect or close to perfect can stay that way without a tremendous effort spent in maintenance. Once you have discovered ritual as a way of allowing community to come to existence, you must remain committed to ritual in order to keep the newly born community alive and prosperous.

Funerals and birth are the two key moments in the individual's journey in community. However private both birth and death look, they are not private, even though the experience does feel intensely personal to the ones experiencing it. From the birthing ritual described in chapter 4, it is clear that in my village life begins in community. The experience of birth reawakens in the community a collective interest in itself, through you. That is, when you are born, the village takes a closer look at its own dynamics to figure out where you fit. In the same way, death spurs the village to take a collective interest because it has lost one of its important members, and therefore death also is an occasion for a lot of collective ritual. The collective mourning is an affirmation that the deceased has left one community and is going to another, and the collective expression of grief and emotion is believed to be the energy that carries the deceased from one realm to another. The community understands that the deceased will continue to serve them as an ancestor, and does all it can to ensure that their spirit makes it safely to their new home.

Perhaps part of the problem that the West has in creating and maintaining community is that people in the West do not remember how to grieve and handle their dead. I described a funeral ritual in great detail in *Of Water and the Spirit* because I realize that funerals and grieving are one area where people in the West have not applied their considerable imagination. The death of someone we love is a real opportunity for our emotional self to become articulated. We are physical entities, but ones that carry a huge load of emotion. We need to begin to imagine how this great part of ourselves can be allowed the space it deserves in the community we are a part of. If we cannot express ourselves emotionally with the members of our own community, something deeply important is missing. And when emotion is missing, usually we are missing as well, unable to be fully present either to ourselves or to one another.

It is deeply important, if people wish to become closer to one another, that they begin to allow the waters of emotion to flow between them. In the West this will mean that men in particular will need to open themselves to the possibility that feeling and expressing emotion are not "feminine" activities, they are human ones. And both men and women will need to be willing to open themselves to the tears of grief, which will begin to make peace with the spirits of the past. This may require a tremendous energy, in order to break away from the prescriptions of tradition, and a huge commitment to healing. But the effort will be well worth it, since such a life-enhancing commitment will serve the greater good of the culture.

CONCLUSION: GIFTS OF INDIGENOUS WISDOM

My work in the West has shown me that the profound longing for that which is missing that Western people express reflects a deep desire for connection. There is a longing for a connection to a sense of purpose and meaning in life that can maintain self-esteem, a desire for a deeper connection to the natural world that we are all a part of, and a desire for an intimate connection with other people who are capable of receiving the unique and individual gifts that each of us has to offer, and hearing the story that each of us has to tell.

The maintenance of these connections in an indigenous culture like that of the Dagara has at its core a spiritual understanding of existence. Beneath the material world that we can see and touch and feel is an energetic world—the world of Spirit—whose vitality enlivens not only all living things, but the very geography of the world that holds life. In the indigenous view, the world of Spirit and the material world coexist; each needs the other because each feeds the other. Without the other, neither is complete. The work of ritual provides the sacred space—the vessel— that we enter with our emotional self, and where the material world and the spiritual world interact. The balance that ritual maintains is health, and the work of ritual is healing. The problems and the disasters of the natural world and the tensions within and between individuals are messages that tell us where the imbalances are, where the healing is needed, and these are messages that we are quite foolish to ignore.

The Dagara creation story says that the planet we are on is a frozen extension of a much brighter and more harmonious spiritual world. If we don't maintain this world, something will happen to the Other World. Our relationship with the Spirit World is a two-way stream, and we need to fine-tune and maintain the lines of communication between the two worlds. The wisdom of the Spirit World offers us guidance, understanding, and healing. Our purpose in this world is linked to a job that returns critical material into the spiritual world. This notion of "As above, so below" is found also in Western lore. The problem is that the imbalances in this world are not being tended to, and this is endangering the health of the Other World. The Dagara people understand that the spirit that animates each one of us in our life can be reborn, and that the purpose of this reincarnation is to try once again to fix this world. And this is why when we come here we are not at peace until we find ourselves useful, wanted, and needed. We do not come to this world on vacation. We come here for service, and we have to remember what that service is. The nature of our service—our purpose—was configured already in the Spirit World before we came here. Community is the mirror that allows us to see our purpose, and the school where we first learn the meaning of service.

The spiritual cosmology of an indigenous people like the Dagara does not involve worship; rather, it is a paradigm for understanding based on careful observation of and a long and intimate relationship with the natural world that surrounds us. The five elements of the Dagara medicine wheel reflect this cosmology, and in symbolic form contain the wisdom of the ancestors. It is my prayer that people in the West will find in this paradigm and the wisdom from which it arises that which is useful to them.

K'a te sankun koro siun a ti tièru
ti kuti ʒumon.
Ka ti tuon gnin a ti vla ʒié ti ti sao déu.

"May all ancestors join force to wake up our spirit
and put good thoughts into our psyche. Then we shall see the good
that awaits us and accept it."

INDEX

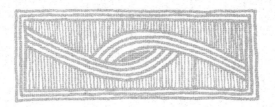

PERMISSIONS

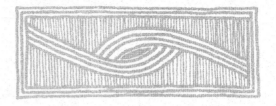

ABOUT THE AUTHOR

Malidoma Patrice Somé, Ph.D., was an initiated man and a gifted diviner from the Dagara tribe of Burkina Faso, West Africa. He was also an incredible teacher, visionary, and healer. In his native language, Malidoma means "be a friend with the stranger."

At the request of his elders, Dr. Somé embarked on a journey to the West to teach the values of his Ancestors. He stood at the threshold between worlds, realities, and mindsets, creating a bridge between the world of his people and the West.

Dr. Somé's books include his renowned autobiography, *Of Water and the Spirit: Ritual, Magic, and Initiation in the Life of an African Shaman,* and *Ritual: Power, Healing and Community*.

For more information about his work, visit Malidoma.com.